LIPPINCOTT
MANUAL *of*
NURSING
PRACTICE
POCKET
GUIDES

Maternal-Neonatal Nursing

D0911104

LIPPINCOTT
MANUAL *of*
NURSING
PRACTICE
POCKET
GUIDES

Maternal-Neonatal Nursing

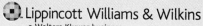
Lippincott Williams & Wilkins
a Wolters Kluwer business
Philadelphia · Baltimore · New York · London
Buenos Aires · Hong Kong · Sydney · Tokyo

STAFF

Executive Publisher
Judith A. Schilling McCann,
RN, MSN

Editorial Director
H. Nancy Holmes

Clinical Director
Joan Robinson, RN, MSN

Senior Art Director
Arlene Putterman

Clinical Project Manager
Beverly Ann Tscheschlog,
RN, BS

Editors
Elizabeth Jacqueline Mills,
Amy Moshier

Clinical Editor
Maryann Foley, RN, BSN

Copy Editors
Kimberly Bilotta (supervisor),
Jane Bradford, Shana
Harrington, Pamela Wingrod

Designer
Matie Anne Patterson
(project manager)

Digital Composition Services
Diane Paluba (manager),
Joyce Rossi Biletz,
Donna S. Morris

Manufacturing
Beth J. Welsh

Editorial Assistants
Megan L. Aldinger,
Karen J. Kirk, Linda K. Ruhf

Design Assistant
Georg W. Purvis IV

Indexer
Barbara Hodgson

**Library of Congress
Cataloging-in-Publication Data**

Maternal-neonatal nursing.
  p. ; cm. — (Lippincott manual of nursing practice pocket guides)
  Includes bibliographical references and index.
  1. Nursing—Handbooks, manuals, etc. I. Lippincott Williams & Wilkins. II. Title. III. Series.
  [DNLM: 1. Maternal-Child Nursing—Handbooks. WY 49 M425 2007]
RT51.M38 2007
618.2'0231—dc22
ISBN 1-58255-907-4 (alk. paper)
                                    2005037921

Contents

Contributors
and consultants

Kimberly Atwood, RN, MSN
Instructor
St. Lukes School of Nursing at Moravian College
Bethlehem, Pa.

Kay Rice Francis, RN, MSN, WHNP
Nursing Instructor
Lake Michigan College
Benton Harbor, Mich.

Shelton M. Hisley, RNC, PhD, WHNP
Senior Associate
Coastline Writing Consultants
Southport, N.C.

Mary-Jo Konkloski, RNC, MSN, ANP-C
Nursing Educator
Arnot Ogden Medical Center
Elmira, N.Y.

Charlotte R. Ledford, RNC, MSN, WHNP
Consultant
Ooltewah, Tenn.

Carol Okupniak, RN, BSN, CCE
Nursing Instructor
Dixon School of Nursing
Abington (Pa.) Memorial Hospital

Luana Rodriguez, ARNP, MSN, CNM
Certified Nurse Midwife
Broward General Medical Center
Fort Lauderdale, Fla.

Elizabeth Simmons-Rowland, RN, MSN, CNS
Assistant Professor, Maternal-Newborn Nursing
Western Carolina University
Candler, N.C.

Ann Triantafillos, RNC, MSN, MEd
Parent & Child Clinical Nurse Specialist
Frederick (Md.) Memorial Healthcare System

Michelle M. Vaughan, RNC, MS, WHNP-C
Lecturer and Clinical Instructor
University of Southern Maine
Portland

Sandra K. Voll, RNC, MS, CNM, FNP, WHNP
Clinical Instructor
Virginia Commonwealth University
    School of Nursing
Richmond

Part one

Disorders

MATERNAL

Abruptio placentae

DESCRIPTION

- Premature separation of the placenta from the uterine wall
- Usually occurs after 20 weeks' gestation, most commonly during the third trimester
- Common cause of bleeding during the second half of pregnancy
- Fetal prognosis variable by gestational age, amount of blood lost, and timing of medical intervention
- Maternal prognosis good if hemorrhage can be controlled
- Classified according to degree of placental separation and severity of maternal and fetal symptoms (see *Degrees of placental separation in abruptio placentae*)
- Also called *placental abruption*
- Possible complications: hemorrhage, shock, renal failure, and disseminated intravascular coagulation (DIC)

PATHOPHYSIOLOGY

- The spontaneous rupture of blood vessels at the placental bed may be caused by a lack of resiliency or by abnormal changes in uterine vasculature.
- The condition may be complicated by hypertension, high multiparity, or by multiple gestation.
- If the bleeding continues unchecked, the placenta may be partially or completely sheared off.

CAUSES

- Exact cause unknown
- Contributing factors:
  - Advanced maternal age
  - Amniocentesis
  - Chronic or gestational hypertension
  - Diabetes mellitus
  - Dietary deficiency

FOCUS IN
DEGREES OF PLACENTAL SEPARATION IN ABRUPTIO PLACENTAE

Mild separation
Internal bleeding between the placenta and the uterine wall characterize mild separation.

Moderate separation
In moderate separation, external hemorrhage occurs through the vagina.

Severe separation
External hemorrhage is also characteristic in severe separation.

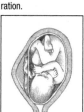
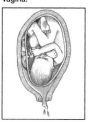
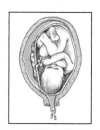

- Multiparity
- Pressure on the vena cava from an enlarged uterus
- Short umbilical cord
- Smoking or cocaine use
- Traumatic injury

ASSESSMENT FINDINGS

Mild abruptio placentae (marginal separation)
- Mild to moderate vaginal bleeding (may not be present)
- Vague lower abdominal discomfort
- Mild to moderate abdominal tenderness
- Fetal monitoring possibly indicating uterine irritability
- Strong and regular fetal heart tones

Moderate abruptio placentae (about 50% placental separation)
- Continuous abdominal pain
- Moderate, dark red vaginal bleeding (may not be present)
- Severe or abrupt onset of symptoms
- Vital signs possibly indicating impending shock

- Tender uterus remaining firm between contractions
- Barely audible or irregular and bradycardic fetal heart sounds
- Labor that usually starts within 2 hours and proceeds rapidly

Severe abruptio placentae (70% placental separation resulting in complete abruption)

- Abrupt onset of agonizing, unremitting uterine pain
- Moderate vaginal bleeding
- Vital signs that indicate rapidly progressive shock
- Absence of fetal heart sounds
- Tender uterus with boardlike rigidity
- Possible increased uterine size in severe concealed abruptions

TEST RESULTS

- Serum hemoglobin level and platelet count are decreased.
- Fibrin split products may reveal DIC and progression of abruptio placentae.
- Pelvic examination under double setup (preparations for an emergency cesarean delivery) and an ultrasound may rule out placenta previa.

TREATMENT

- Assessment, control, and restoration of lost blood
- Delivery of a viable neonate
- Prevention of coagulation disorders
- If placental separation is severe with no signs of fetal life, induction of vaginal delivery unless contraindicated by uncontrolled hemorrhage or other complications

  ALERT Because of possible fetal blood loss through the placenta, a pediatric team should be ready at delivery to assess and treat the neonate for shock, blood loss, and hypoxia.

  ALERT Complications of abruptio placentae require prompt appropriate treatment. With a complication such as DIC, the patient needs immediate intervention with platelets and whole blood, as ordered, to prevent exsanguination.

- Withholding of oral liquids and solids until delivery of the fetus
- Maintaining the patient on bed rest until delivery
- Administration of I.V. fluid infusion (by large-bore catheter) as ordered
- Initiation of cesarean delivery for maternal or fetal distress

KEY PATIENT OUTCOMES

The patient will:
- maintain stable vital signs
- maintain balanced fluid volume
- express feelings of increased comfort
- communicate feelings about the situation
- use available support systems to aid in coping
- give birth to a viable neonate.

NURSING INTERVENTIONS

- Insert an indwelling urinary catheter, and monitor intake and output.
- Obtain blood samples for hemoglobin level and hematocrit, coagulation studies, and type and crossmatching, as ordered.
- Provide emotional support during labor.
- Provide information on progress and condition of the fetus during labor.
- Encourage the patient to verbalize her feelings.
- Help the patient develop effective coping strategies.
- Give I.V. fluids and blood products.
- Monitor maternal vital signs, including central venous pressure.
- Assess for vaginal bleeding.
- Institute electronic monitoring of fetal heart rate.
- Monitor uterine contractions for frequency, intensity, and resting tone.
- Monitor the progression of labor.
- Refer the patient for professional counseling, if indicated before discharge.

PATIENT TEACHING

Be sure to cover:
- the disorder, diagnosis, and treatment
- signs of placental abruption
- possibility of an emergency cesarean delivery
- possibility of the delivery of a premature infant
- changes to expect in the postpartum period
- possibility of neonatal death
- factors affecting survival of neonate
- importance of frequent monitoring and prompt management to reduce risk of maternal or fetal death.

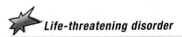

Life-threatening disorder

Amniotic fluid embolism

DESCRIPTION

- Escape of amniotic fluid into maternal circulation
- Results from a defect in the amniotic membranes after rupture or from partial abruptio placentae
- Risk of possible deposition of meconium, lanugo, and vernix in fetal pulmonary arterioles

PATHOPHYSIOLOGY

- An open maternal uterine blood sinus occurs as a result of a defect in the membranes or after membrane rupture or partial premature separation.
- Amniotic fluid is forced into the open sinus.
- Solid particles then enter maternal circulation and travel to the lungs, leading to pulmonary embolism.

CAUSES

- Believed to be an anaphylactoid type of response
- Predisposing factors: intrauterine fetal death, high parity, abruptio placentae, oxytocin augmentation, and advanced maternal age

ASSESSMENT FINDINGS

- Sudden dyspnea
- Increasing restlessness and anxiety
- Tachypnea
- Chest pain
- Coughing with pink, frothy sputum
- Hemorrhage
- Cyanosis
- Shock disproportionate to blood loss

TEST RESULTS

■ Arterial blood gas levels show hypoxemia.
■ D-dimer level is elevated.
■ Lung ventilation-perfusion scan shows a ventilation-perfusion mismatch.
■ Chest X-rays show a possible small infiltrate or effusion.

TREATMENT

■ Administration of oxygen, blood, and heparin
■ Insertion of a central venous pressure line
■ Close monitoring of cardiopulmonary status
■ Immediate delivery of the neonate

▶ **COLLABORATION** *Caring for the patient with an amniotic fluid embolism requires maximizing oxygenation, maintaining cardiopulmonary function and hemodynamic status, and reducing oxygen demand with rest and activity restrictions. In addition, the fetus must be delivered quickly to minimize risks associated with decreased placental perfusion secondary to the drop in blood pressure. The multidisciplinary care required by this patient and her fetus might include members of the intensive care unit (ICU), a surgeon (for insertion of the central venous catheter, if indicated), and a neonatologist and members of the neonatal ICU.*

KEY PATIENT OUTCOMES

The patient will:
■ maintain adequate ventilation
■ maintain adequate cardiac output
■ maintain a patent airway
■ verbalize feelings of increased comfort
■ give birth to a viable neonate.

NURSING INTERVENTIONS

■ Know that the prognosis of the mother and fetus depends on the size of the embolism, fetal gestational age, and the skill and speed of the emergency interventions.

- Administer oxygen via face mask or cannula, as ordered, and assess vital signs continuously for changes.
- Anticipate the need for endotracheal intubation.
- Monitor fetal heart rate patterns continuously.
- Prepare to initiate cardiopulmonary resuscitation.
- Arrange to transfer the patient to the ICU, and prepare for immediate cesarean delivery.
- Assess the patient for signs and symptoms of disseminated intravascular coagulation, which may develop from the presence of particles in the bloodstream.
- Administer fibrinogen, as ordered.

PATIENT TEACHING

Time for patient teaching may be limited because of the seriousness of her condition. However, be sure to cover:
- the disorder, diagnosis, and treatment
- procedures being done
- medications being administered
- signs and symptoms to report to health care providers.

Cardiac disease
DESCRIPTION

- Involves some type of impaired cardiac function
- Greater incidence of pregnancy in women with cardiac disease as a result of advances in cardiac treatments
- Pregnancy risk variable by type and extent of patient's disease (see *Cardiac disease and pregnancy*)

PATHOPHYSIOLOGY

- The underlying problem depends on the location and severity of the cardiac disorder.
- Valvular stenosis decreases blood flow through the valve, increasing the workload on heart chambers located before the stenotic valve.
- Insufficiency permits blood to leak through an incompletely closed valve, increasing the workload on heart chambers on either side of the affected valve.

CARDIAC DISEASE AND PREGNANCY

A patient with cardiac disease may experience a difficult pregnancy; a successful outcome for both mother and fetus depends on the type and extent of the disease. A patient with a class I or a class II condition usually completes a successful pregnancy and delivery without major complications. A woman in class III must maintain complete bed rest to complete the pregnancy. A patient in class IV is a poor candidate for pregnancy.

Class	Description
I	The patient has no restrictions on physical activity. Ordinary activity causes no discomfort, cardiac insufficiency, or angina.
II	The patient has a slight limitation on physical activity. Ordinary activity causes excessive fatigue, palpitations, dyspnea, or angina.
III	The patient has a moderate to marked limitation on activity. With less than ordinary activity, she experiences excessive fatigue, palpitations, dyspnea, or angina.
IV	The patient can't engage in any physical activity without discomfort. Cardiac insufficiency or angina occurs even at rest.

■ The normal heart can compensate for increased demands, but if myocardial or valvular disease develops, or if the patient has a congenital heart defect, cardiac decompensation may occur.

ALERT *A patient with a cardiac disorder is at greatest risk when hemodynamic changes reach their maximum, between the 28th and 32nd weeks of gestation.*

CAUSES

■ Congenital heart disease, such as atrial septal defect, ventricular septal defect, pulmonary stenosis, or coarctation of the aorta
■ Rheumatic heart disease leading to endocarditis with scar-tissue formation on the mitral, aortic, or tricuspid valves, with resulting stenosis or insufficiency

ASSESSMENT FINDINGS

■ Dyspnea
■ Tachycardia

- Fatigue
- Orthopnea
- Edema of hands, face, and feet
- Palpitations
- Diastolic murmur at the heart's apex
- Cough
- Hemoptysis
- Crackles at the bases of the lungs

TEST RESULTS

- Electrocardiography (ECG) reveals cardiac changes in the mother.
- Echocardiography reveals cardiomegaly.
- Late decelerations on a fetal monitor are possible if the mother's cardiac decompensation has caused placental insufficiency and incompetency.
- Ultrasonography may show fetal growth restriction.

TREATMENT

▶ **COLLABORATION** *Caring for the pregnant woman with cardiac disease requires a multidisciplinary approach. A cardiologist will monitor her cardiac status. Depending on the degree of compromise, respiratory and physical therapy and nutritional therapy may be necessary. In addition, a neonatologist will be involved during labor and birth, and a perinatologist may be consulted during the antepartal, intrapartal, and postpartal periods. Social services may be necessary to provide home care during the pregnancy and after birth of the neonate.*

- Close medical supervision with more frequent prenatal visits and adjustments in prepregnancy drug therapy
- Rest
- Limited sodium and increased protein and iron intake
- Prophylactic antibiotic as indicated
- Serial ultrasounds, nonstress tests, and biophysical profile to evaluate fetal status
- Prophylactic antibiotic therapy during labor for women with mitral valve prolapse to protect the valve

KEY PATIENT OUTCOMES

The patient will:
- maintain adequate cardiac output and placental perfusion
- maintain hemodynamic stability
- perform activities of daily living within limitations of disease
- maintain adequate fluid balance
- maintain adequate ventilation
- give birth to a viable neonate.

NURSING INTERVENTIONS

- Assess maternal vital signs and cardiopulmonary status closely for changes.
- Question the patient about increasing shortness of breath, cough, dyspnea, palpitations, or edema.
- Monitor fetal heart rate for changes.
- Monitor weight gain throughout pregnancy.
- Assess the patient for edema, noting any evidence of pitting.
- Reinforce the use of prescribed medications.
- Alert the patient to danger signs and symptoms that should be reported immediately.
- Reinforce the need for more frequent prenatal visits, and assist with arranging follow-up testing.
- Anticipate the need for increased doses of maintenance medications, and explain the rationale for this increase.
- Assess the patient's nutritional pattern; work with her to develop a workable meal plan that's high in protein and iron.
- Stress the need for prenatal vitamins and stool softeners, if ordered.
- Encourage frequent rest periods throughout the day, with activity pacing and energy-conservation measures.
- Advise the patient to report any signs and symptoms of infection, such as upper respiratory tract or urinary tract infection, as soon as noticed.
- Advise the patient to rest in the lateral recumbent position; if necessary, use the semi-Fowler position.
- Prepare the patient for labor, anticipating the use of epidural anesthesia, low forceps during the second stage of labor, and continuous ECG monitoring.
- During labor, closely monitor fetal heart rate, uterine contractions, and maternal vital signs for changes.
- Assess the patient's vital signs closely after delivery.

- Anticipate anticoagulant and cardiac glycoside therapy for the patient with severe heart failure immediately after delivery.
- Encourage ambulation, as ordered, as soon as possible after delivery.
- Anticipate administration of a prophylactic antibiotic, if not already ordered, after delivery.

PATIENT TEACHING

Be sure to cover:
- the disorder, diagnosis, and treatment, including dietary program
- danger signs and symptoms indicating a worsening of her condition and the need to notify the physician
- need for weighing self daily and checking for edema
- medication dosages, administration, potential adverse effects, and monitoring needs
- need to adhere to scheduled follow-up prenatal visits
- measures to decrease fatigue.

Cephalopelvic disproportion
DESCRIPTION

- Narrowing of the birth canal
- Disproportion between the size of the normal fetal head and the pelvic diameters
- Results in failure to progress in labor

PATHOPHYSIOLOGY

- In primigravidas, the fetal head normally engages between 36 to 38 weeks' gestation.
- When this event occurs before labor begins, it's assumed that the pelvic inlet is adequate.
- When the fetal head engages or proves it fits into the pelvic brim, it's likely that it will also be able to pass through the midpelvis and through the outlet.
- In multigravidas, the fetal head usually engages when labor begins; previous vaginal delivery of a full-term neonate without problems is substantial proof that the birth canal is adequate.

- With cephalopelvic disproportion (CPD), the fetus's head doesn't engage.
- The head remains a floating entity, possibly resulting in malpositioning, further complicating the condition.
- If membranes rupture, the possibility of cord prolapse greatly increases.

CAUSES

- Size of the patient's pelvis (major contributing factor)
- Inlet contraction (occurs when the narrowing of the anteroposterior diameter is less than 11 cm or the maximum transverse diameter is 12 cm or less; may result from maternal pelvic fracture, malformation, or small size)
- Outlet contraction (narrowing of the transverse diameter [located at the distance between the ischial tuberosities] at the outlet to less than 11 cm; can also be a contributing factor)

ASSESSMENT FINDINGS

- Lack of fetal head engagement in a primigravida due to a fetal abnormality, such as a larger-than-usual head, or a pelvic abnormality, such as a smaller-than-usual pelvis

TEST RESULTS

- Anteroposterior diameter measures less than 11 cm, and the maximum transverse diameter is 12 cm or less (inlet contraction).
- Transverse diameter at outlet is less than 11 cm.
- Ultrasonography reveals a larger-than-usual fetal head.

TREATMENT

- If the pelvic measurements (especially the inlet measurement) are borderline or just adequate, and the fetal lie and position are good: possible trial labor to determine whether labor can progress normally
- If descent of the presenting part and dilation of the cervix are occurring: possible continuation of trial labor
- If labor doesn't progress or complications develop: cesarean delivery

KEY PATIENT OUTCOMES

The patient will:
- progress through labor without complications or evidence of fetal distress
- deliver a viable neonate vaginally or by cesarean delivery.

NURSING INTERVENTIONS

- Instruct the primiparous patient to maintain her prenatal visit schedule.
- Monitor the progress of trial labor; if, after 6 to 12 hours, adequate progress in labor can't be documented or if fetal distress occurs, prepare the patient for cesarean delivery.
- Remember that it may be difficult for the patient to undertake a labor if she knows cesarean delivery is essential.
- Be alert to the patient's feelings about trial labor; she may express self-consciousness or the perception that she's being judged.
- If dilation doesn't occur, the patient may feel discouraged and inadequate if she believes herself to be responsible for perceived "failure."
- Allow the patient to verbalize her feelings and beliefs related to being needlessly subjected to pain.
- If the trial labor fails and cesarean delivery is scheduled, explain why it's necessary.
- Provide support for the patient's family, who may feel frightened and helpless when a problem occurs in labor and delivery.
- Explain that cesarean delivery isn't an inferior birth method; remind the patient and her family that it will facilitate a successful outcome for both mother and neonate.

PATIENT TEACHING

Be sure to cover:
- the disorder, diagnosis, and treatment
- necessary monitoring techniques
- steps involved in a trial labor
- cesarean delivery, including indications for it in this situation
- postcesarean delivery care.

Cervical insufficiency

DESCRIPTION

- Painless premature dilation of the cervix
- Generally occurs at 16 to 20 weeks' gestation, most commonly around 20 weeks
- Also called *premature cervical dilation* or *incompetent cervix*

PATHOPHYSIOLOGY

- A weak, structurally defective cervix spontaneously dilates.
- Contractions are absent.
- Continued cervical dilation leads to rupture of membranes, release of amniotic fluid, and uterine contractions, ultimately leading to the delivery of the fetus, commonly before viability.

CAUSES

- Associated with congenital structural defects or previous cervical trauma resulting from surgery or delivery
- Associated also with increasing maternal age and increased uterine volume, such as from hydramnios or multiple gestations
- May result from in utero exposure secondary arising from the mother's use of diethylstilbestrol

ASSESSMENT FINDINGS

- History of one or more second trimester spontaneous abortions
- Cervical dilation in the absence of contractions or pain
- Pink-stained vaginal discharge or amniotic fluid
- Increased pelvic pressure with possible ruptured membranes and release of amniotic fluid

TEST RESULTS

- Ultrasonography reveals defect or cervical shortening.
- A nitrazine test may indicate rupture of membranes.

TREATMENT

- Placement of a purse-string suture, called a *cerclage*, in the cervix to help keep it closed until term or until the patient goes into labor
- Bed rest after surgery
- Removal of sutures at predetermined time of gestation
- Emotional support

KEY PATIENT OUTCOMES

The patient will:
- maintain bed rest
- express feelings about her condition
- exhibit no signs or symptoms of labor
- maintain pregnancy until term with delivery of a viable neonate.

NURSING INTERVENTIONS

- Assess complaints of vaginal drainage, and investigate the patient's history for previous cervical surgeries.
- Prepare the patient for cervical cerclage under regional anesthesia, as indicated; monitor maternal vital signs and fetal heart rate patterns closely.
- Instruct the patient about signs and symptoms of pregnancy danger and about signs and symptoms of labor; explain the need to notify her health care provider should these signs occur.
- Maintain bed rest after surgery, as ordered; if necessary, place the patient in a slight or modified Trendelenburg position.
- Encourage follow-up.
- Advise the patient that the sutures will be removed before delivery at a time determined by her health care provider.

PATIENT TEACHING

Be sure to cover:
- the disorder, diagnosis, and treatment
- signs and symptoms of labor and the need to notify the health care provider
- necessary activity restrictions or limitations
- need to adhere to scheduled follow-up prenatal visits.

Diabetes mellitus

DESCRIPTION

- Metabolic disorder characterized by hyperglycemia (elevated serum glucose level) resulting from lack of insulin, lack of insulin effect, or both
- Disorder of carbohydrate, protein, and fat metabolism
- Four general classifications (see *Classification of diabetes*)
- Increased risk of congenital anomalies, hydramnios, macrosomia, gestational hypertension, spontaneous abortion, and fetal death with type 1 diabetes
- Risk of developing diabetes mellitus in 1 to 25 years: 30% to 40% for women with gestational diabetes

PATHOPHYSIOLOGY

- In people genetically susceptible to type 1 diabetes, a triggering event causes a production of autoantibodies against the beta cells of the pancreas.
  - The resulting destruction of the beta cells leads to a decline in and ultimate lack of insulin secretion.
  - Insulin deficiency leads to hyperglycemia, enhanced lipolysis (decomposition of fat), and protein catabolism.
  - These characteristics occur when more than 90% of the beta cells have been destroyed.
- Type 2 diabetes mellitus is a chronic disease caused by one or more of the following factors: impaired insulin production, inappropriate hepatic glucose production, or peripheral insulin receptor insensitivity.
  - Genetic factors are significant.

CLASSIFICATION OF DIABETES

The Expert Committee on the Diagnosis and Classification of Diabetes Mellitus (2003) has identified the four following classifications:

- type 1: absolute insulin insufficiency
- type 2: insulin resistance or deficiency
- impaired fasting glucose and impaired glucose tolerance: hyperglycemia at lower level than qualifying as diabetes and without the symptoms of diabetes
- gestational diabetes: glucose intolerance due to pregnancy.

  – Onset is accelerated by obesity and a sedentary lifestyle.
  – Added stress can be a pivotal factor.
■ Gestational diabetes mellitus occurs when a patient not previously di-
  agnosed with diabetes shows glucose intolerance during pregnancy.
■ It isn't known whether gestational diabetes results from an inadequate
  insulin response to carbohydrates, excessive insulin resistance, or
  both.
■ Risk factors for gestational diabetes include obesity, history of deliver-
  ing large neonates (usually more than 10 lb [4.5 kg]), unexplained fetal or perinatal loss, evidence of congenital anomalies in previous
  pregnancies, age (older than age 25), and family history of diabetes.

CAUSES

■ Environment (infection, diet, toxins, and stress)
■ Heredity
■ Lifestyle changes in genetically susceptible people

ASSESSMENT FINDINGS

■ Hyperglycemia
■ Glycosuria
■ Polyuria
■ Increased incidence of candidal infections
■ Hydramnios
■ Signs and symptoms of macrovascular and microvascular changes,
  such as peripheral vascular disease, retinopathy, nephropathy, and
  neuropathy

TEST RESULTS

■ Oral glucose challenge test reveals an increased fasting plasma glucose
  level. (See *Oral glucose challenge test values for pregnancy.*)
■ Two abnormal levels or a fasting glucose level greater than 105 mg/dl
  may reveal diabetes mellitus.

ORAL GLUCOSE CHALLENGE TEST VALUES FOR PREGNANCY

If the results of a blood glucose screening test are abnormal, a 3-hour glucose challenge test (GCT) is done. A diagnosis of gestational diabetes mellitus (GDM) can be made only after an abnormal GCT. Normal values for a GCT are:

- fasting blood glucose level less than 105 mg/dl
- level less than 190 mg/dl at 1 hour
- level less than 165 mg/dl at 2 hours
- level less than 145 mg/dl at 3 hours.

According to the guidelines of the American Diabetes Association (2004), two or more abnormal values confirm a diagnosis of GDM.

TREATMENT

▷ *COLLABORATION Multidisciplinary care is necessary for the pregnant woman with diabetes. An endocrinologist may be needed to assist with controlling blood glucose levels. Nutritional therapy is indicated to assist with dietary needs and planning. A diabetes educator can be valuable in helping the patient learn how to manage her condition. In addition, social services can help with identifying financial and community resources as well as assist with arranging home care follow-up.*

Gestational diabetes mellitus

- Blood glucose level monitoring; fasting blood sugar (FBS) and 2-hour postprandial
- Target glucose levels for FBS less than 100 mg and postprandial less than 120 mg
- Careful monitoring of diet, exercise, and insulin administration and patient education

↖ *ALERT Oral antidiabetics are contraindicated during pregnancy because of their adverse effects on the fetus and neonate; however, these agents may be used in the second or third trimester if the patient is noncompliant with her insulin regimen.*

Type 1 diabetes mellitus
■ Close monitoring of glucose levels because of the tendency for wide
  fluctuations
■ In general, insulin requirements decrease during the first trimester and
  increase during the second and third trimesters
■ Evaluation of glycosylated hemoglobin levels every 3 months as an
  overall indicator of blood glucose control

KEY PATIENT OUTCOMES

The patient will:
■ maintain blood glucose levels within acceptable parameters
■ verbalize understanding of the disorder and treatment needs during
  pregnancy
■ demonstrate adherence to the treatment plan
■ remain free from infection and complications
■ give birth to a viable neonate.

NURSING INTERVENTIONS

■ Monitor the patient's status carefully throughout the pregnancy; assess
  weight gain, blood glucose levels, nutritional intake, and fetal growth
  parameters.
■ Review results of fingerstick blood glucose monitoring; assess the patient for signs and symptoms of hypoglycemia and hyperglycemia.
■ Assist with arranging follow-up laboratory studies, including glycosylated hemoglobin levels and urine studies, as necessary.
■ Encourage a consistent exercise program, including the use of snacks.
■ Assist with preparations for labor, including explanations about possi-
  ble labor induction and required monitoring.
■ Closely assess the patient in the postpartum period for changes in
  blood glucose levels and insulin requirements.
  – Typically the patient with preexisting diabetes will require no in-
    sulin in the immediate postpartum period (because insulin resis-
    tance is gone) and will return to her prepregnancy insulin require-
    ments within several days.
  – The patient with gestational diabetes usually exhibits normal blood
    glucose levels within 24 hours after delivery, requiring no further
    insulin or diet therapy.

■ Encourage the patient with gestational diabetes to adhere to follow-up health maintenance visits to obtain glucose testing for possible type 2 diabetes.

PATIENT TEACHING

Be sure to cover:
■ the disorder, diagnosis, and treatment
■ insulin preparation and administration, if appropriate
■ nutritional regimen
■ fingerstick blood glucose monitoring (technique and frequency)
■ signs and symptoms of hypoglycemia and hyperglycemia and when to notify the health care provider
■ activity and exercise restrictions
■ need to adhere to scheduled follow-up visits and tests.

Dysfunctional labor

DESCRIPTION

■ Sluggishness in the force of labor (contractions)
■ Prolonged labor as a result
■ Also called *inertia*

PATHOPHYSIOLOGY

■ Dysfunctional labor can occur at any point in labor but is generally classified as *primary* or *secondary.*
■ Primary dysfunctional labor occurs at the onset of labor.
■ Secondary dysfunctional labor occurs later in labor.
■ The incidence of maternal postpartum infection and hemorrhage and neonatal mortality is higher in women who have prolonged labors than in those who don't.

CAUSES

■ Problems related to passenger: fetal malposition, malpresentation, or unusually large size
■ Problems related to passage: pelvic contractures

TYPES OF CONTRACTIONS

Below are illustrations of the different uterine activity types. Depending on your
assessment, you may need to intervene to promote adequate labor contractions.

Typical contractions
Typical uterine contractions occur every 2 to 5 minutes during active labor and
typically last 30 to 90 seconds.

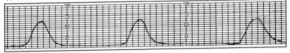

Hypotonic contractions
Hypotonic contractions are accompanied by a rise in pressure of no more than
10 mm Hg during each contraction.

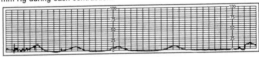

Hypertonic contractions
Hypertonic contractions don't allow the uterus to rest between contractions, as
shown by a resting pressure of 40 to 50 mm Hg.

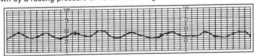

- Problems related to power: hypotonic, hypertonic, or uncoordinated
  uterine contractions (see *Types of contractions*)
- Medications, such as analgesics or anesthetics, given too early during
  labor
- Other conditions, such as a distended bladder or bowel

ASSESSMENT FINDINGS

Hypotonic contractions
- Most common during the active phase; results in protraction of this
  phase
- Number of contractions usually low or infrequent.

- Contractions commonly limited to two or three in a 10-minute period
- Pattern highly irregular and typically doesn't cause pain
- Resting tone of the uterus below 10 mm Hg
- Strength of contractions below 25 mm Hg

Hypertonic contractions

- Most common during the latent phase; results in protraction of this phase
- Intensity of contractions similar to hypotonic contractions
- Tend to occur frequently
- Marked by an increase in resting tone to more than 15 mm Hg
- Patient complaints of pain

Uncoordinated contractions

- Occur erratically
- Lack of regular pattern; interferes with the patient's ability to rest or use breathing techniques between contractions

TEST RESULTS

- Ultrasonography reveals fetal malposition, an unusually large fetus, or pelvic contractures.
- Uterine monitoring reveals hypotonic, hypertonic, or uncoordinated contractions.

TREATMENT

Hypotonic contractions

- Inducement or augmentation of labor, if contractions are too weak or infrequent to be effective
- Inducement of labor if the cervix deemed ready for dilation, as evidenced by a score of 8 on the cervical readiness scale (see *Evaluating cervical readiness*, page 24)
- Inducement of labor if the fetus is in danger or if labor doesn't occur spontaneously and the fetus appears to be at term
- Cervical ripening via stripping of membranes or application of prostaglandin gel or laminaria before induction of labor
- Oxytocin

EVALUATING CERVICAL READINESS

Bishop's score is a tool you can use to assess whether a woman is ready for labor. A score ranging from 0 to 3 is given for each of five factors: cervical dilation, length (effacement), station, consistency, and position. If the woman's score exceeds 8, the cervix is considered suitable for induction.

Scoring factor	Score			
	0	1	2	3
Dilation (cm)	0	1 to 2	3 to 4	3 to 4
Effacement (%)	0 to 30	40 to 50	60 to 70	80
Station	−3	−2	−1 to 0	+1 to +2
Consistency	Firm	Medium	Soft	
Position	Posterior	Mild position	Anterior	

Adapted with permission from Bishop, E.H. "Pelvic Scoring for Elective Induction," *Obstetrics and Gynecology* 24:266, 1964.

Hypertonic contractions

- Rest with analgesia (such as morphine sulfate), and possible inducement of sedation
- Comfort measures (changing the linens and the mother's gown, darkening room lights, and decreasing noise and stimulation)
- Cesarean delivery (if the fetal heart rate (FHR) decelerates, the first stage of labor is abnormally long, or progress isn't made with pushing [second-stage arrest])

Uncoordinated contractions

- Oxytocin administration
- Discontinuation of oxytocin if hypertension occurs

Problems with passage or passenger

- If the pelvic measurements (especially the inlet measurement) are borderline or just adequate, and the fetal lie and position are good: possible trial labor

- If descent of the presenting part and dilation of the cervix are occurring: possible continuation of labor
- If labor doesn't progress or if complications develop: cesarean delivery

KEY PATIENT OUTCOMES

The patient will:

- exhibit a more coordinated uterine contraction pattern
- progress through labor without complications or evidence of fetal distress
- give birth to a viable neonate vaginally or by cesarean delivery.

NURSING INTERVENTIONS

- Explain the events to the patient and her family; explain that the contractions are ineffective.
- Provide comfort measures, including nonpharmacologic pain relief.
- Continuously monitor uterine contractions and FHR patterns.
- Offer fluids as appropriate; institute I.V. therapy.
- Assist with measures to induce or augment labor; monitor oxytocin infusion, if used.
- Encourage frequent voiding.

PATIENT TEACHING

Be sure to cover:

- the disorder, diagnosis, and treatment
- necessary monitoring techniques
- pain relief measures
- medications for augmenting labor, including possible adverse effects
- steps involved in a trial labor, if appropriate
- cesarean delivery, including indications
- postcesarean delivery care.

Ectopic pregnancy

DESCRIPTION

- Implantation of a fertilized ovum outside the uterine cavity, most commonly in the fallopian tube (see *Implantation sites of ectopic pregnancy*)
- Good maternal prognosis with prompt diagnosis, appropriate surgical intervention, and control of bleeding
- Poor fetal prognosis (rare incidence of survival to term with abdominal implantation)
- About 33% chance of giving birth to a live neonate in a subsequent pregnancy
- Incidence: about 1 of 200 pregnancies in whites; about 1 of 120 pregnancies in nonwhites
- Complications: rupture of fallopian tube, hemorrhage, shock, peritonitis, infertility, disseminated intravascular coagulation, and death

PATHOPHYSIOLOGY

- Transport of a blastocyst to the uterus is delayed.
- The blastocyst implants at another available vascularized site, usually the fallopian tube lining.
- Normal signs of pregnancy are initially present.
- Uterine enlargement occurs in about 25% of cases.
- Human chorionic gonadotropin (hCG) hormonal levels are lower than in uterine pregnancies.
- If not interrupted, internal hemorrhage occurs with rupture of the fallopian tube.

CAUSES

- Congenital defects in the reproductive tract
- Diverticula
- Ectopic endometrial implants in the tubal mucosa
- Endosalpingitis
- Intrauterine device
- Previous surgery, such as tubal ligation or resection
- Sexually transmitted tubal infection
- Transmigration of the ovum
- Tumors pressing against the tube

IMPLANTATION SITES OF ECTOPIC PREGNANCY

In about 95% of patients with ectopic pregnancy, the ovum implants in part of the fallopian tube: the fimbria, ampulla, or isthmus. Other possible abnormal sites of implantation include the interstitium, ovarian ligament, ovary, abdominal viscera, and internal cervical os.

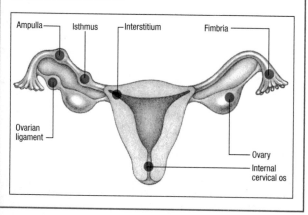

ASSESSMENT FINDINGS

- Amenorrhea
- Abnormal menses (after fallopian tube implantation)
- Slight vaginal bleeding
- Unilateral pelvic pain over the mass
- If fallopian tube ruptures, sharp lower abdominal pain, possibly radiating to the shoulders and neck

ALERT *Ectopic pregnancy sometimes produces symptoms of normal pregnancy or no symptoms other than mild abdominal pain (especially in abdominal pregnancy), making diagnosis difficult.*

- Possible extreme pain when cervix is moved and adnexa palpated
- Boggy and tender uterus
- Possible enlargement of adnexa

TEST RESULTS

- Serum hCG level is abnormally low; when repeated in 48 hours, the level remains lower than the levels found in a normal intrauterine pregnancy.
- Realtime ultrasonography may show an intrauterine pregnancy or ovarian cyst.
- Culdocentesis shows free blood in the peritoneum.
- Laparoscopy may reveal a pregnancy outside the uterus.

TREATMENT

- Initially, in the event of pelvic-organ rupture, management of shock
- Diet determined by clinical status
- Activity determined by clinical status
- Transfusion with whole blood or packed red blood cells
- Broadspectrum I.V. antibiotics
- Supplemental iron
- Methotrexate (Rheumatrex)
- Laparotomy and salpingectomy if culdocentesis shows blood in the peritoneum; possibly after laparoscopy to remove affected fallopian tube and control bleeding
- Microsurgical repair of the fallopian tube for patients who wish to have children
- Oophorectomy for ovarian pregnancy
- Hysterectomy for interstitial pregnancy
- Laparotomy to remove the fetus for abdominal pregnancy

KEY PATIENT OUTCOMES

The patient will:
- have stable vital signs
- express feelings about the current situation
- use available support systems to aid in coping.

NURSING INTERVENTIONS

- Determine the date and description of the patient's last menstrual period.
- Monitor vital signs for changes.

- Assess vaginal bleeding, including amount and characteristics.
- Assess pain level.
- Monitor intake and output.
- Assess for signs of hypovolemia and impending shock.
- Prepare the patient with excessive blood loss for emergency surgery.
- Administer prescribed blood transfusions and analgesics.
- Provide emotional support.
- Administer Rh_o(D) immune globulin (RhoGAM), as ordered, if the patient is Rh negative.
- Provide a quiet, relaxing environment.
- Encourage the patient to express feelings of fear, loss, and grief.
- Help the patient develop effective coping strategies.
- Refer the patient to a mental health professional, if necessary, prior to discharge.

PATIENT TEACHING

Be sure to cover:
- the disorder, diagnosis, and treatment
- postoperative care
- prevention of recurrent ectopic pregnancy
- prompt treatment of pelvic infections
- risk factors for ectopic pregnancy, including surgery involving the fallopian tubes and pelvic inflammatory disease.

 Life-threatening disorder

Gestational hypertension
DESCRIPTION

- High blood pressure (greater than 140 mm Hg systolic or 90 mm Hg diastolic) not accompanied by proteinuria, most commonly occurring after the 20th week of gestation in a nulliparous patient
- High risk of fetal mortality because of the increased incidence of premature delivery, placental abruption, and intrauterine growth restriction
- Among the most common causes of maternal death in developed countries (especially with complications)
- Occurrence in about 7% of pregnancies and commonly in lower socioeconomic groups

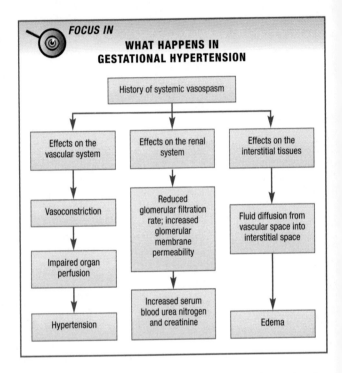

FOCUS IN

WHAT HAPPENS IN GESTATIONAL HYPERTENSION

History of systemic vasospasm

Effects on the vascular system	Effects on the renal system	Effects on the interstitial tissues
Vasoconstriction	Reduced glomerular filtration rate; increased glomerular membrane permeability	Fluid diffusion from vascular space into interstitial space
Impaired organ perfusion		
Hypertension	Increased serum blood urea nitrogen and creatinine	Edema

- Preeclampsia (elevated blood pressure with proteinuria) occurring after the 20th week of gestation; may be mild or severe
- Eclampsia (preeclampsia with seizures) occurring between the 24th week of gestation and the end of the first postpartum week
- Roughly 5% incidence of preeclampsia progressing to eclampsia
- Possible complications: abruptio placentae, coagulopathy, stillbirth, seizures, coma, premature labor, renal failure, maternal hepatic damage, and hemolysis, elevated liver enzyme levels, low platelet count (HELLP syndrome)
- Formerly called *pregnancy-induced hypertension*

PATHOPHYSIOLOGY

- Generalized arteriolar vasospasm is thought to cause decreased blood flow through the placenta and maternal organs.

■ This leads to intrauterine growth restriction, placental infarcts, and abruptio placentae. (See *What happens in gestational hypertension.*)

CAUSES

■ Exact cause unknown
■ Contributing factors:
  - Autoimmune disease
  - Autointoxication
  - Autolysis of placental infarcts
  - Chronic hypertension
  - Chronic renal disease
  - Diabetes
  - Geographic, ethnic, racial, nutritional, immunologic, and familial factors
  - Maternal age (younger than age 19 or older than age 35)
  - Maternal sensitization to total proteins
  - Preexisting vascular disease
  - Pyelonephritis
■ Risk factors: first-time pregnancy, multiple fetuses, obesity, and a history of vascular disease

ASSESSMENT FINDINGS

■ Sudden weight gain
■ Irritability
■ Emotional tension
■ Severe frontal headache
■ Blurred vision, scotomata
■ Epigastric pain or heartburn
■ Severe preeclampsia: blood pressure of 160/110 mm Hg or higher
■ Generalized edema, especially of the face
■ Pitting edema of the legs and feet
■ Hyperreflexia
■ Oliguria
■ Vascular spasm, papilledema, retinal edema or detachment, and arteriovenous nicking or hemorrhage (seen on ophthalmoscopy)
■ Seizures

TEST RESULTS

- Proteinuria of more than 300 mg/24 hours (1+ on dipstick) reveals preeclampsia.
- Proteinuria of 5 g/24 hours (3+) or more reveals severe eclampsia.
- Hemolysis, elevated liver enzymes, and a decreased platelet count reveals HELLP syndrome.
- Serial ultrasonography evaluates fetal well-being and the amniotic fluid volume.
- Nonstress tests and biophysical profiles evaluate fetal well-being.

TREATMENT

COLLABORATION Gestational hypertension affects multiple body systems and requires a multidisciplinary approach to care. Medical and nursing health care providers focus on administering medications to treat hypertension and prevent potential complications. Nutritional consultation may be necessary to help with lifestyle changes involving diet. If the patient experiences preeclampsia or eclampsia, neurologists or renal specialists may also be needed. Social services may be consulted for a referral for home-care evaluation and follow-up.

- Measures to halt progression of the disorder and ensure fetal survival
- Prompt labor induction, especially if the patient is near term (38 weeks' gestation; advocated by some clinicians)
- Adequate nutrition; limited caffeine and low-sodium diet, if indicated
- Complete bed rest, preferably in the left lateral supine position
- Antihypertensives
- Magnesium sulfate
- Oxytocin administration, if indicated
- Oxygen
- Possible cesarean delivery

KEY PATIENT OUTCOMES

The patient will:
- maintain normal vital signs
- maintain adequate fluid volume
- avoid complications
- remain oriented to the environment

EMERGENCY INTERVENTIONS FOR GESTATIONAL HYPERTENSION

When caring for a patient with gestational hypertension, be prepared to perform the following interventions:

- Observe for signs of fetal distress by closely monitoring results of stress and nonstress tests.
- Keep emergency resuscitative equipment and anticonvulsants at hand in case of seizures and cardiac or respiratory arrest.
- Carefully monitor magnesium sulfate administration. Signs of drug toxicity include absence of patellar reflexes, flushing, muscle flaccidity, decreased urinary output, significant blood pressure drop (> 15 mm Hg), and a respiratory rate of fewer than 12 breaths/minute. Keep calcium gluconate at the bedside to counteract the toxic effects of magnesium sulfate.
- Prepare for emergency cesarean delivery, if indicated. Alert the anesthesiologist and pediatrician.
- To protect the patient from injury, maintain seizure precautions. Don't leave a patient with unstable blood pressure unattended. Maintain a patent airway, and have supplemental oxygen readily available.

- give birth to a viable neonate by vaginal or cesarean delivery.

NURSING INTERVENTIONS

- Assess maternal vital signs and fetal heart rate frequently; monitor for changes in blood pressure, pulse rate, respiratory rate, fetal heart rate, vision, level of consciousness, deep tendon reflexes, episgastric or abdominal pain, and headache unrelieved by medication. Report changes immediately.
- Give prescribed drugs. (See *Emergency interventions for gestational hypertension.*)

ALERT *When magnesium sulfate is ordered, always administer the drug as a piggyback infusion so that the drug can be discontinued immediately if the patient develops signs and symptoms of toxicity. Obtain a baseline serum magnesium level before initiating therapy, and monitor levels frequently after administration is initiated. Keep in mind that to be effective as an anticonvulsant, serum magnesium levels should be between 5 and 8 mg/dl. Levels above 8 mg/dl indicate toxicity.*

- Monitor extent of edema and degree of pitting.
- Encourage elevation of edematous arms or legs.
- Eliminate constricting clothing, hose, slippers, and bed linens.
- Monitor daily weights and intake and output.
- Assist with or insert an indwelling urinary catheter, if necessary.
- Provide a quiet, darkened room.
- Encourage compliance with bed rest.
- Provide emotional support, encouraging the patient to express her feelings.
- Help the patient develop effective coping strategies.

PATIENT TEACHING

Be sure to cover:
- the disorder, diagnosis, and treatment
- signs and symptoms of preeclampsia and eclampsia
- importance of bed rest in the left lateral position, as ordered
- adequate nutrition and a low-sodium diet
- good prenatal care
- control of preexisting hypertension
- early recognition and prompt treatment of preeclampsia.

Gestational trophoblastic disease
DESCRIPTION

- Developmental anomaly of the placenta that converts the chorionic villi into a mass of clear fluid-filled vesicles
- Two types of moles
  - Complete moles: neither an embryo nor an amniotic sac
  - Partial mole: embryo (usually with multiple anomalies) and amniotic sac (see *Comparing complete and partial moles*)
- Major cause of second trimester bleeding
- Also called *molar pregnancy* or *hydatidiform mole*

ALERT Early detection of gestational trophoblastic disease is essential because it's associated with choriocarcinoma, a fast-growing, highly invasive malignancy.

COMPARING COMPLETE AND PARTIAL MOLES

Gestational trophoblastic disease may be classified as a complete or partial mole based on chromosomal analysis.

A complete mole is characterized by swelling and cystic formation of all trophoblastic cells. No fetal blood is present. If an embryo did develop, it was most likely only 1 to 2 mm in size and died early on. A complete mole is highly associated with the development of choriocarcinoma.

A partial mole is characterized by edema of a layer of the trophoblastic villi with some of the villi forming normally. Fetal blood may be present in the villi, and an embryo up to the size of 9 weeks' gestation may be present. Typically, a partial mole has 69 chromosomes in which there are three chromosomes for every one pair.

PATHOPHYSIOLOGY

- Trophoblastic villi cells located in the outer ring of the blastocyst (the structure that develops via cell division around 3 to 4 days after fertilization) rapidly increase in size, begin to deteriorate, and fill with fluid.
- The cells become edematous, appearing as grapelike clusters of vesicles.
- As a result, the embryo fails to develop past the early stages.

CAUSES

- Exact cause unknown
- May be associated with poor maternal nutrition (specifically, an insufficient intake of protein and folic acid), a defective ovum, chromosomal abnormalities, or hormonal imbalances
- Preceding molar pregnancy in about 50% of patients with choriocarcinoma
- Preceding spontaneous or induced abortion, ectopic pregnancy, or normal pregnancy in the remaining 50% of patients

ASSESSMENT FINDINGS

- Disproportionate enlargement of the uterus; possible grapelike clusters noted in vagina on pelvic examination
- Excessive nausea and vomiting; abdominal cramping
- Intermittent or continuous bright red or brownish vaginal bleeding

- Passage of tissue resembling grapelike clusters
- Symptoms of gestational hypertension before 20 weeks' gestation
- Absence of fetal heart tones

TEST RESULTS

- Radioimmunoassay of human chorionic gonadotropin (hCG) levels reveals extremely elevated levels for early pregnancy.
- Histologic examination may reveal the presence of vesicles.
- Ultrasonography performed after 3 months' gestation reveals grapelike clusters rather than a fetus, an absence of fetal skeleton, and evidence of a snowstorm-like pattern.
- Hemoglobin level, hematocrit, red blood cell (RBC) count, prothrombin time, partial thromboplastin time, fibrinogen levels, and hepatic and renal function findings are all abnormal.
- White blood cell count and erythrocyte sedimentation rate are increased.

TREATMENT

- Suction and curettage, if indicated
- Weekly monitoring of beta-hCG levels until normal for 3 consecutive weeks
- Periodic follow-up for 1 to 2 years
- Pelvic examinations and chest X-rays at regular intervals
- Emotional support
- Avoidance of pregnancy until hCG levels are normal (may take up to 1 year)

KEY PATIENT OUTCOMES

The patient will:
- have stable vital signs
- express her feelings
- use available support systems to aid in coping
- adhere to the follow-up schedule
- remain free from complications.

NURSING INTERVENTIONS

- Obtain baseline vital signs.
- Preoperatively, observe the patient for signs of complications, such as hemorrhage, uterine infection, and vaginal passage of vesicles.
- Save any expelled tissue for laboratory analysis.
- Prepare the patient physically and emotionally for surgery, if indicated.
- Postoperatively, monitor vital signs and fluid intake and output, and assess for signs of hemorrhage.
- Encourage the patient and her family to express their feelings.
- Offer emotional support, and help them through the grieving process.
- Help the patient and her family develop effective coping strategies, referring them to a mental health professional, if needed.

PATIENT TEACHING

Be sure to cover:
- the disorder, diagnosis, and treatment
- importance of adhering to follow-up testing and visits
- signs and symptoms of possible complications
- contraception and avoidance of pregnancy.

Human immunodeficiency virus infection
DESCRIPTION

- Causative organism for acquired immunodeficiency syndrome
- Sexually transmitted infection
- Possible serious implications for patient and fetus
- Also known as *HIV*

PATHOPHYSIOLOGY

- HIV infection is caused by a retrovirus that targets the helper T lymphocytes that contain the CD4$^+$ antigen. (See *How HIV replicates*, page 38.)
- The virus integrates itself into the cell's genetic makeup, ultimately causing cellular dysfunction.
- The cells are no longer able to mount an appropriate immune response, leaving the patient vulnerable to opportunistic infections.

FOCUS IN

HOW HIV REPLICATES

This flowchart shows the steps in human immunodeficiency virus (HIV) cell replication.

HIV enters the bloodstream.

↓

HIV attaches to the surface of the CD4+ T lymphocyte.

↓

Proteins on the HIV cell surface bind to the protein receptors on the host cell's surface.

↓

HIV penetrates the host cell membrane and injects its protein coat into the host cell's cytoplasm.

↓

HIV's genetic information, ribonucleic acid (RNA), is released into the cell after its protective coat is partially dissolved.

↓

The single-stranded viral RNA, via the action of reverse transcriptase, is converted (transcribed) into double-stranded deoxyribonucleic acid (DNA).

↓

Viral DNA integrates itself into the host cell's nucleus.

↓

Integrase, an enzyme, inserts HIV's double-stranded DNA into the host cell's DNA.

→

When the host cell is activated, the viral DNA takes over, telling the host cell to produce RNA (now viral RNA).

↓

Two strands of RNA are produced and transported out of the nucleus.

↓

One strand becomes the subunits of the HIV (that is, enzymes and structural proteins); the other becomes the genetic material for new viruses.

↓

Cleavage occurs (viral subunits are separated) through the action of protease, a viral enzyme.

↓

HIV subunits combine to make up new viral particles and begin to break down the host cell membrane.

↓

The genetic material in the new viral particles merges with the cell membrane that has been changed, forming a new viral envelope (outer covering).

↓

Viral budding occurs, in which the new HIV is released to enter the circulation.

CAUSES

- Human immunodeficiency virus
- May be contracted through sexual intercourse, exposure to infected blood, vertical transmission across the placenta to the fetus during pregnancy, labor and delivery, birth, or by breast milk ingested by the neonate

ASSESSMENT FINDINGS

- Lymphadenopathy
- Bacterial pneumonia
- Dermatologic problems
- Diarrhea
- Fatigue
- Fevers
- Nausea, anorexia
- Night sweats
- Memory loss, headaches
- Thrush
- Thrombocytopenia
- Severe vaginal yeast infection unresponsive to treatment
- Abnormal Papanicolaou test
- Frequent human papillomavirus infections, frequent and recurrent bacterial vaginosis, trichomonas, and genital herpes infections
- Weight loss

TEST RESULTS

- Western blot test confirms two positive enzyme-linked immunosorbent assays.
- CD4+ T-lymphocyte count is less than 200 cells/μl.

TREATMENT

COLLABORATION *Caring for the pregnant patient with HIV requires a multidisciplinary approach. An immunologist or infectious disease specialist may be needed to assist in guiding therapy. A nutritional specialist may be necessary to ensure adequate nutrition for the mother and for fetal growth and develop-*

ment. Infection control specialists may be helpful in minimizing the risk for infection transmission. Additionally, a mental health specialist can be enlisted to assist with the emotional repercussions of HIV. Social services can assist with referrals for community services and support groups, financial concerns, and follow-up in the home.

- Combination antiretroviral therapy in an attempt to reduce the mother's viral load, thus minimizing the risk of vertical transmission of the infection to the fetus
- Supportive care

KEY PATIENT OUTCOMES

The patient will:
- achieve management of symptoms
- demonstrate use of protective measures
- verbalize understanding of safe sex practices
- use available support systems for coping
- remain free from complications
- demonstrate adherence to the treatment plan and therapy
- give birth to a viable neonate.

NURSING INTERVENTIONS

ALERT Institute standard precautions in caring for the patient throughout the pregnancy and after delivery, and when caring for the neonate.

- Teach the patient measures to minimize the risk of virus transmission.
- Provide emotional support and guidance for the patient who is HIV-positive and considering pregnancy.
- Allow the patient who has recently received a diagnosis of HIV infection to verbalize her feelings; provide support.
- Monitor CD4+ T-lymphocyte counts and viral loads, as indicated.
- Assess the patient for signs and symptoms of opportunistic infections.
- Encourage the patient to comply with prenatal follow-up visits.
- Administer antiretroviral therapy as ordered.
- Instruct the patient in medication therapy, and assist with scheduling medication administration.
- Evaluate the patient for compliance on return visits.

ALERT *Institute measures during labor and delivery to minimize the fetus's risk of exposure to maternal blood or body fluids. Avoid use of internal fetal monitors, scalp blood sampling, forceps, and vacuum extraction to prevent the creation of an open lesion of the fetal scalp.*

- Advise the mother that breast-feeding isn't recommended because of the risk of possible virus transmission.
- Withhold blood sampling and injections of the neonate until maternal blood has been removed with the first bath.

PATIENT TEACHING

Be sure to cover:
- the disorder, diagnosis, and treatment
- modes of transmission
- adherence to medication regimen
- importance of informing potential sexual partners, caregivers, and health care providers of HIV infection status
- signs and symptoms of impending infection and importance of seeking immediate medical care
- safer sex practices
- infection control measures.

Hyperemesis gravidarum
DESCRIPTION

- Severe and unremitting nausea and vomiting that begins in the first trimester and persists after the first trimester
- Common with first pregnancy and with conditions that produce high levels of human chorionic gonadotropin (hCG), such as gestational trophoblastic disease or multiple gestations

PATHOPHYSIOLOGY

- Elevated levels of hCG are present in all patients during early pregnancy; the level usually declines after 12 weeks, corresponding to the usual duration of morning sickness.
- In hyperemesis gravidarum, the hCG levels are commonly higher and

remain higher beyond the first trimester, possibly in association with *Helicobacter pylori* infection.

- Decreased fluid intake and prolonged vomiting cause dehydration.
- Dehydration increases the serum concentration of hCG, which, in turn, exacerbates the nausea and vomiting.

CAUSES

- Linked to trophoblastic activity, gonadotropin production, and psychological factors
- Possible causes:
  - Biliary tract disease
  - Changes in gastrointestinal motility
  - Decreased gastric motility
  - Decreased secretion of free hydrochloric acid in the stomach
  - Drug toxicity
  - Hypofunction of the anterior pituitary and adrenal cortex
  - Inflammatory obstructive bowel disease
  - Pancreatitis (elevated serum amylase levels are common)
  - Psychological factors (in some cases)
  - Thyroid dysfunction
  - Transient hyperthyroidism
  - Vitamin deficiency (especially of B_6)

ASSESSMENT FINDINGS

- Unremitting nausea and vomiting (cardinal sign)
- Vomitus usually containing undigested food, mucus, and small amounts of bile initially, progressing to containing only bile and mucus and, finally, blood and material resembling coffee grounds
- Reports of substantial weight loss and eventual emaciation
- Thirst
- Hiccups
- Oliguria
- Vertigo
- Headache
- Electrolyte imbalance
- Dehydration
- Metabolic acidosis
- Jaundice
- Pallor

TEST RESULTS

- Serum protein, chloride, sodium, and potassium levels are decreased.
- Blood urea nitrogen levels are increased.
- Hemoglobin levels are elevated.
- White blood cell count is elevated.
- Ketonuria and slight proteinuria are present.
- Radiologic studies may indicate molar or twin pregnancy.

TREATMENT

COLLABORATION The patient with hyperemesis gravidarum typically requires multidisciplinary care. A nutritional specialist can develop a meal plan that ensures adequate intake for the patient and supports fetal growth and development. If psychological factors are contributing to the patient's condition, a referral to a mental health professional may be necessary. Additionally, social services can provide assistance in home management activities, especially if there are other children at home.

- Restoration of fluid and electrolyte balance with I.V. fluid therapy
- Control of vomiting with an antiemetic

ALERT No drug has been approved by the Food and Drug Administration for the treatment of nausea and vomiting during pregnancy. If an antiemetic is prescribed, it is done so with caution and the benefits must outweigh the risk to the patient and fetus.

- Maintenance of adequate nutrition and rest
- Progression of diet to oral feedings as tolerated (clear liquid diet, then a full liquid diet and, finally, small, frequent meals of high-protein solid foods); if necessary, total parenteral nutrition

KEY PATIENT OUTCOMES

The patient will:

- exhibit a decrease in the episodes of nausea and vomiting
- remain free from signs and symptoms of dehydration and electrolyte imbalance
- maintain a stable weight without additional losses

- demonstrate consumption of adequate nutrition to support self and pregnancy
- verbalize feelings related to the current situation and use positive coping strategies
- give birth to a viable neonate.

NURSING INTERVENTIONS

- Administer I.V. fluids, as ordered, until the patient can tolerate oral feedings.
- Monitor fluid intake and output, vital signs, skin turgor, daily weight, serum electrolyte levels, and urine ketone levels; anticipate the need for electrolyte replacement therapy.
- Provide frequent mouth care.
- Consult a dietitian or nutritionist to provide a diet high in dry, complex carbohydrates, and for suggestions to control nausea (such as vitamin B_6 supplementation or use of ginger root).
- Suggest company, diversionary conversation, and decreased liquid intake at mealtimes.
- Instruct the patient to remain upright for 45 minutes after eating.
- Suggest that the patient eat a high-protein snack at night and recommend eating two or three dry crackers on awakening in the morning, before getting out of bed.
- Advise patient to wait 1 hour after eating to consume fluids.
- Provide reassurance and a calm, restful atmosphere.
- Encourage the patient to discuss her feelings about her pregnancy and the disorder.
- Help her develop effective coping strategies.
- Assist with protective measures to conserve energy and promote rest, including relaxation techniques, moderate exercise (if tolerated), and activities to prevent fatigue.

PATIENT TEACHING

Be sure to cover:
- the disorder, diagnosis, and treatment
- possible contributing factors
- nutritional needs and planning
- energy conservation measures

- measures to control nausea and vomiting, including medication therapy, as appropriate
- signs and symptoms of complications and the importance of reporting them immediately.

Isoimmunization

DESCRIPTION

- Rh-negative patient carrying an Rh-positive fetus
- Risk of hemolytic disease in the neonate, if untreated
- Formerly a major cause of kernicterus and neonatal death (prognosis improved with use of $Rh_0(D)$ immune globulin [RhoGAM])
- Also known as *Rh sensitivity*

PATHOPHYSIOLOGY

- With isoimmunization, an antigen-antibody immunologic reaction within the body occurs when an Rh-negative pregnant patient carries an Rh-positive fetus.
- During the Rh-negative patient's first pregnancy, she becomes sensitized by exposure to Rh-positive fetal blood antigens inherited from the father.
- A patient may also become sensitized through blood transfusions with alien Rh antigens, from inadequate doses of $Rh_0(D)$, or from failure to receive $Rh_0(D)$ after significant fetal-maternal leakage from abruptio placentae.
- Subsequent pregnancy with an Rh-positive fetus provokes increasing amounts of maternal agglutinating antibodies to cross the placental barrier, attach to Rh-positive cells in the fetus, and cause hemolysis and anemia.
- To compensate for this, the fetus steps up the production of red blood cells (RBCs), and erythroblasts (immature RBCs) appear in the fetal circulation.
- Extensive hemolysis results in the release of large amounts of unconjugated bilirubin, which the liver can't conjugate and excrete, thereby causing hyperbilirubinemia and hemolytic anemia. (See *Pathogenesis of Rh isoimmunization*, page 46.)

FOCUS IN

PATHOGENESIS OF RH ISOIMMUNIZATION

Rh isoimmunization spans pregnancies in Rh-negative mothers who give birth to Rh-positive neonates. The illustrations below outline the process of isoimmunization.

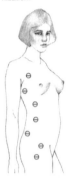

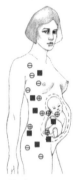

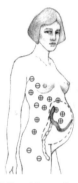

1. Before pregnancy, the woman has Rh-negative blood.

2. She becomes pregnant with an Rh-positive fetus. Normal antibodies appear.

3. Placental separation occurs.

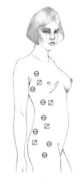

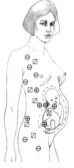

4. After delivery, the mother develops anti–Rh-positive antibodies.

5. With the next Rh-positive fetus, antibodies enter fetal circulation, causing hemolysis.

KEY:
Rh– blood ⊕
Rh+ blood ⊖
Normal antibodies ■
Anti-Rh antibodies ☑

CAUSES

- Rh-negative mother sensitized to Rh-positive antigens on first pregnancy
- Subsequent pregnancies with Rh-positive fetuses

ASSESSMENT FINDINGS

- None (mother shows no symptoms)

TEST RESULTS

- Increased concentration (optical density) of bilirubin and RBC breakdown products in the amniotic fluid may reveal isoimmunization.
- Anti-D antibody titer of 1:16 or greater may reveal isoimmunization.
- Radiologic studies may reveal edema and, in those with hydrops fetalis, the halo sign (edematous, elevated, subcutaneous fat layers) and the Buddha position (fetus's legs crossed).

TREATMENT

- Monitoring of the indirect Coombs' test or to −1
- Delta optical density analysis of amniotic fluid at 26 weeks' gestation
- Intrauterine transfusion
- Possible early delivery
- Administration of $Rh_o(D)$ immunoglobulin at 28 weeks' gestation and within 72 hours following delivery of Rh-positive neonate to attain passive antibody protection for future pregnancies

KEY PATIENT OUTCOMES

The patient will:
- verbalize understanding of the disorder and its treatment
- demonstrate adequate coping measures
- give birth to a viable neonate.

NURSING INTERVENTIONS

- Assess all pregnant patients for possible Rh incompatibility.
- Expect to administer RhoGAM after transfusion reaction, ectopic pregnancy, or spontaneous or induced abortion. Other indications include

placenta previa, abruptio placentae during the second or third trimester, and amniocentesis results that confirm isoimmunization. (See *Administering RhoGAM*, page 208.)

- Administer RhoGAM as ordered to Rh-negative women at 28 weeks' gestation and within 72 hours after delivery, as ordered.
- Assist with intrauterine transfusion as indicated.
- Beforehand IU transfusion, obtain a baseline fetal heart rate (FHR) by electronic monitoring; explain the procedure and its purpose to the patient.
- After the transfusion, carefully observe the patient for uterine contractions, amniotic fluid leaking from the vagina, and fluid leakage from the puncture site.
- Monitor FHR for tachycardia, bradycardia, or variable decelerations.
- Prepare the patient for a planned delivery, usually 2 to 4 weeks before term date, depending on maternal history, serologic tests, and amniocentesis results.
- Assist with induction of labor, if indicated.
- During labor, monitor the fetus electronically for oxygen saturation.
- Indication of fetal distress necessitates immediate cesarean delivery.
- Provide emotional support to the patient and her family.

PATIENT TEACHING

Be sure to cover:
- the disorder, diagnosis, and treatment
- procedures used to determine sensitization, including preprocedure and postprocedure care
- need for follow-up
- RhoGAM administration
- plans for delivery, possibly before term due date.

Multiple gestation
DESCRIPTION

- Pregnancy involving more than one fetus
- Considered a complication (effects caused by presence of multiple fetuses)
- Also called *multiple pregnancy*

PATHOPHYSIOLOGY

- Multiple gestations are the result of the fertilization of one ova that divides into two or more zygotes or the fertilization of two or more ova.
- The increasing use of fertility drugs has lead to a rise in the number of multiple gestations.

CAUSES

- Heredity (in cases of natural dizygotic [fraternal] twins)
- Use of fertility drugs
- Contributing factors: multiparity and increased maternal age

ASSESSMENT FINDINGS

- Increase in size of uterus at a rate faster than usual
- Complaints of feeling fluttering actions at different areas of the abdomen rather than at one specific, consistent spot
- Amount of fetal activity greater than expected for gestation stage
- Multiple sets of fetal heart sounds
- Increased fatigue and backache

TEST RESULTS

- Alpha-fetoprotein levels are elevated.
- Ultrasonography reveals more than one gestational sac.

TREATMENT

- Close maternal and fetal monitoring and surveillance
- Immediate management of possible complications, such as gestational hypertension, gestational diabetes, hydramnios, placenta previa, preterm labor and birth, anemia, postpartum bleeding, and twin-to-twin transfusion

KEY PATIENT OUTCOMES

The patient will:
- verbalize understanding of her condition
- remain free from signs and symptoms of possible complications

- demonstrate positive coping strategies
- give birth to viable neonates as close to term as possible.

NURSING INTERVENTIONS

- Inform the patient about the condition and the need for close, frequent follow-up.
- Encourage frequent rest periods throughout the day.
- Urge the patient to rest in the side-lying position.
- Monitor maternal vital signs, weight gain, and fundal height at every visit; assess fetal heart rates and position at every visit.
- Arrange for follow-up testing, such as ultrasound and nonstress tests.
- Urge the patient to take prenatal vitamins and to eat a well-balanced diet high in vitamins and iron.
- Alert the patient of the signs and symptoms that might indicate preterm labor or other complications and the need to report these to her health care provider immediately.
- Provide emotional support to the patient and her family.
- Allow the patient to verbalize her fears and anxieties.
- Correct any misconceptions that the patient voices.
- During labor, provide separate electronic fetal monitoring for each fetus.
- Be alert for hypotonic contractions, which might necessitate labor augmentation or cesarean delivery.
- At delivery, gather enough equipment and medications to care for each neonate.
- Ensure that nurses are available for each neonate and for the mother during delivery.
- Monitor patient closely after delivery for signs and symptoms of postpartum hemorrhage.

PATIENT TEACHING

Be sure to cover:
- the condition, diagnosis, and treatment
- need for adequate rest and nutrition
- importance of close, frequent follow-up throughout pregnancy
- signs and symptoms necessitating notification of the health care provider
- possibility of preterm birth or need for cesarean delivery.

Oligohydramnios

DESCRIPTION

- Severe reduction of amniotic fluid volume (typically less than 500 ml at term); highly concentrated fluid
- Possibility of prolonged, dysfunctional labor (usually beginning before term)
- Fetal risks: renal anomalies, pulmonary hypoplasia, hypoxia, increased skeletal deformities, and wrinkled, leathery skin

PATHOPHYSIOLOGY

- Normally, when the fetal kidneys begin to function, the fetus urinates into the amniotic fluid.
- Fetal urine becomes the major source of amniotic fluid.
- Oligohydramnios occurs when the fetus is unable to make urine or the passage of urine is blocked, leading to a decrease in amniotic fluid.

CAUSES

- Exact cause unknown
- Any condition that prevents the fetus from making urine or that blocks urine from going into the amniotic sac
- Contributing factors: uteroplacental insufficiency, premature rupture of membranes prior to labor onset, maternal hypertension, maternal diabetes, intrauterine growth restriction, postterm pregnancy, fetal renal agenesis, polycystic kidneys, and urinary tract obstructions

ASSESSMENT FINDINGS

- Asymptomatic
- Lagging fundal height growth

TEST RESULTS

- Ultrasonography reveals no pockets of amniotic fluid larger than 1 cm.

TREATMENT

- Close medical supervision of the mother and fetus
- Fetal monitoring
- Amnioinfusion (infusion of warmed sterile normal saline or lactated Ringer's solution) to treat or prevent variable decelerations during labor

KEY PATIENT OUTCOMES

The patient will:
- maintain stable vital signs, weight, and fluid balance
- demonstrate understanding of the condition and its treatment
- remain free from complications associated with amnioinfusion
- demonstrate adequate coping mechanisms
- give birth to a viable neonate.

NURSING INTERVENTIONS

- Monitor maternal and fetal status closely, including vital signs and fetal heart rate patterns.
- Monitor maternal weight gain pattern, notifying the health care provider if weight loss occurs.
- Provide emotional support before, during, and after ultrasonography.
- Inform the patient about coping measures if fetal anomalies are suspected.
- Instruct her about signs and symptoms of labor, including those she'll need to report immediately.
- Reinforce the need for close supervision and follow-up.
- Assist with amnioinfusion as indicated.
- Encourage the patient to lie on her left side.
- Ensure that amnioinfusion solution is warmed to body temperature.
- Continuously monitor maternal vital signs and fetal heart rate during the amnioinfusion procedure.
- Note the development of any uterine contractions, notify the health care provider, and continue to monitor closely.
- Maintain strict sterile technique during amnioinfusion.

  ALERT *Watch for continuous fluid drainage from the vagina, and report any sudden cessation of fluid flow, which suggests fetal head engagement leading to fluid retention within the uterus and possible development of hydramnios.*

PATIENT TEACHING

Be sure to cover:

- the disorder, diagnosis, and treatment
- the importance of daily fetal activity monitoring
- signs and symptoms of impending labor and the need to notify the health care provider
- the amnioinfusion procedure, including preprocedure and postprocedure care
- complications associated with amnioinfusion.

Placenta previa

DESCRIPTION

- Placental implantation in the lower uterine segment, encroaching on the internal cervical os
- Common cause of bleeding during the second half of pregnancy (among patients who develop placenta previa during the second trimester, less than 15% have persistent previa at term)
- Occurs about 1 in every 200 pregnancies, more commonly after age 35; more common in multigravidas than in primigravidas
- Good maternal prognosis if hemorrhage can be controlled
- Preterm delivery possible with heavy bleeding
- Fetal prognosis variable by gestational age and amount of blood loss (risk for death is greatly reduced by frequent monitoring and prompt management)

PATHOPHYSIOLOGY

- The placenta covers all or part of the internal cervical os. (See *Three types of placenta previa*, page 54.)

FOCUS IN
THREE TYPES OF PLACENTA PREVIA

The degree of placenta previa depends largely on the extent of cervical dilation at the time of examination because the dilating cervix gradually uncovers the placenta, as shown below.

Marginal placenta previa
If the placenta covers just a fraction of the internal cervical os, the patient has marginal, or low-lying, placenta previa.

Partial placenta previa
The patient has the partial, or incomplete, form of the disorder if the placenta caps a larger part of the internal os.

Total placenta previa
If the placenta covers all of the internal os, the patient has total, complete, or central placenta previa. This type is associated with greater blood loss.

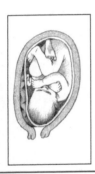
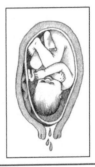
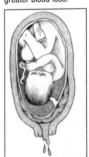

CAUSES

- Exact cause unknown
- Contributing factors:
  - Advanced maternal age (older than age 35)
  - Defective vascularization of the decidua
  - Endometriosis
  - Factors that may affect the site of placental attachment to the uterine wall
  - Multiparity
  - Multiple gestation
  - Previous uterine surgery
  - Smoking

ASSESSMENT FINDINGS

- Onset of painless, bright red, vaginal bleeding after 20 weeks' gestation
- Vaginal bleeding before onset of labor, typically episodic and stopping spontaneously
- May be asymptomatic
- Soft, nontender uterus
- Fetal malpresentation
- Minimal descent of fetal presenting part
- Good fetal heart sounds

TEST RESULTS

- Maternal hemoglobin level is decreased.
- Kleihauer Betke in Rh-negative mother may indicate the presence of fetal blood cells from fetomaternal hemorrhage greater than 30 ml.
- Transvaginal ultrasonography determines placental position.
- Pelvic examination is contraindicated.

ALERT *Pelvic examination isn't commonly performed because it increases maternal bleeding and can dislodge more of the placenta.*

TREATMENT

- Maternal stabilization and fetal monitoring
- Control of blood loss; blood replacement
- Delivery of viable neonate
- Prevention of coagulation disorders
- With fetus of less than 36 weeks' gestation, careful observation to determine safety of continuing pregnancy or need for preterm delivery
- Hospitalization with complete bed rest until 36 weeks' gestation with complete placenta previa
- Possible vaginal delivery, with minimal bleeding or rapidly progressing labor

ALERT *Because of possible significant blood and resulting fetal and neonatal hypovolemia, shock, and hypoxemia, a neonatal/pediatric team should be on hand during delivery to immediately assess, resuscitate, and stabilize the neonate. The neonate may also require a blood transfusion.*

- Nothing by mouth initially, then as guided by clinical status
- Bed rest
- I.V. fluids, using a large-bore catheter
- Immediate cesarean delivery in severe hemorrhage or at 36 weeks' gestation

KEY PATIENT OUTCOMES

The patient will:
- maintain stable vital signs
- maintain normal fluid volume
- express feelings of increased comfort
- verbalize her feelings and concerns about her condition
- use available support systems to aid coping.
- give birth to a viable neonate as close to term as possible, vaginally or by cesarean delivery.

NURSING INTERVENTIONS

- If continuation of the pregnancy is deemed safe for patient and fetus, administer magnesium sulfate as ordered for premature labor.
- Obtain blood samples for complete blood count and blood type and crossmatching.
- Institute complete bed rest.
- If the patient with placenta previa is experiencing active bleeding, continuously monitor her blood pressure, pulse rate, respirations, central venous pressure, intake and output, and amount of vaginal bleeding as well as the fetal heart rate and rhythm.
- Assist with application of intermittent or continuous electronic fetal monitoring as indicated by maternal and fetal status.
- Have oxygen readily available for use should fetal distress occur, as indicated by bradycardia, tachycardia, late or variable decelerations, pathologic sinusoidal pattern, unstable baseline, or loss of variability.
- If the patient is Rh-negative and not sensitized, administer $Rh_o(D)$ immune globulin (RhoGAM) after every bleeding episode.
- Administer prescribed I.V. fluids and blood products.
- Provide information about labor progress and the condition of the fetus.

- Prepare the patient and her family for a possible cesarean delivery and the birth of a preterm neonate, and provide thorough instructions for postpartum care.
- If the fetus is less than 36 weeks' gestation, expect to administer an initial dose of betamethasone; explain that additional doses may be given again in 24 hours and, possibly, for the next 2 weeks to help mature the neonate's lungs.
- Explain that the fetus' survival depends on gestational age and amount of maternal blood loss. Request consultation with a neonatologist or pediatrician to discuss a treatment plan with the patient and her family.
- Assure the patient that frequent monitoring and prompt management greatly reduce the risk of neonatal death.
- Encourage the patient and her family to verbalize their feelings, help them to develop effective coping strategies, and refer them for counseling, if necessary.
- Anticipate the need for a referral for home care if the patient's bleeding ceases and she's to return home on bed rest.
- During the postpartum period, monitor the patient for signs of early and late postpartum hemorrhage and shock.

PATIENT TEACHING

Be sure to cover:
- the disorder, diagnosis, and treatment
- signs and symptoms of placenta previa
- possibility of emergency cesarean delivery
- possibility of the birth of a premature neonate or of fetal or neonatal demise
- postpartum physical and emotional changes.

Polyhydramnios

DESCRIPTION

- Abnormally large amount of amniotic fluid in the uterus
- Normal range from 500 to 1,000 ml at term; typically greater than 2,000 ml in polyhydramnios at 40 weeks' gestation

- Possible complications: prolapsed umbilical cord when membranes rupture, increased incidence of malpresentations, increased perinatal mortality from fetal malformations and premature deliveries, and increased incidence of postpartum maternal hemorrhage
- Also called *hydramnios*

PATHOPHYSIOLOGY

- Normally, amniotic fluid volume is maintained by a balance of fetal fluid production (lung liquid and urine) and fluid resorption (fetal swallowing and flow across the membrane to the fetus or the maternal uterus).
- Fetal urine is the primary source of amniotic fluid with output at term ranging from 400 to 1,200 ml/day.
- Fetal swallowing is believed to be the major route of amniotic fluid resorption.
- With polyhydramnios, fluid accumulates because of a problem with the fetus's ability to swallow or absorb the fluid or as a result of overproduction of urine.
- Fluid may have increased gradually (chronic type) by the third trimester or rapidly (acute type) between 20 and 24 weeks' gestation.

CAUSES

- Exact cause unknown in about 35% of all cases
- May be associated with diabetes mellitus (about 25%), erythroblastosis (about 10%), multiple gestations (about 10%), anomalies of the central nervous system (such as neural tube defects), or GI anomalies such as tracheoesophageal fistula that prevent ingestion of the amniotic fluid (about 20%)

ASSESSMENT FINDINGS

- Depend on the length of gestation, the amount of amniotic fluid, and whether the disorder is chronic or acute
- Mild signs and symptoms: maternal abdominal discomfort, slight dyspnea, and edema of feet and ankles
- Severe signs and symptoms: severe dyspnea, orthopnea, and significant edema of the vulva, legs, and abdomen

- Symptoms common to mild and severe cases: uterine enlargement greater than expected for the length of gestation, and difficulty in outlining the fetal parts and in detecting fetal heart sounds

TEST RESULTS

- Ultrasonography shows evidence of excess amniotic fluid as well as underlying conditions.
- Amniotic fluid index is 20 cm or greater.

TREATMENT

- High-protein, low-sodium diet
- Mild sedation
- Indomethacin (Indocin) to decrease fetal urine production and amniotic fluid
- Amniocentesis to remove excess fluid and decrease pressure on uterine wall
- Induction of labor if the fetus is mature and symptoms are severe

KEY PATIENT OUTCOMES

The patient will:
- maintain stable vital signs, weight, and fluid balance
- demonstrate understanding of the condition and its treatment
- remain free from complications associated with amniocentesis
- demonstrate adequate coping mechanisms
- give birth to a viable neonate.

NURSING INTERVENTIONS

- Maintain bed rest.
- Monitor the patient for signs and symptoms of premature labor.
- Encourage the patient to avoid straining on defecation.
- Immediately report any complaints of increasing dyspnea.
- Monitor maternal vital signs and fetal heart rate frequently; report changes immediately.
- Prepare the patient for amniocentesis and possible labor induction, as appropriate; keep in mind that amniocentesis for fluid removal is only temporary and may need to be done repeatedly.

PATIENT TEACHING

Be sure to cover:
- the disorder, diagnosis, and treatment
- signs and symptoms of impending labor and the need to notify the health care provider
- amniocentesis procedure, including preprocedure and postprocedure care
- complications associated with amniocentesis and condition
- neonatal care.

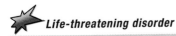
Life-threatening disorder

Postpartum hemorrhage

DESCRIPTION

- Uterine blood loss greater than 500 ml
- Early postpartum hemorrhage: blood loss during the first 24 hours after delivery
- Late postpartum hemorrhage: blood loss after the first postpartum day, anytime during the remaining 6-week postpartum period (most common 7 to 14 days after delivery)
- Predisposing factors: delivery of a large neonate, multiple gestation, hydramnios, dystocia, grand multiparity, trauma during delivery, and medications used during labor or surgery

PATHOPHYSIOLOGY

- Normally, after a vaginal delivery, a blood loss of up to 500 ml is considered acceptable; for a cesarean delivery, the acceptable range for blood loss is typically 1,000 to 1,200 ml.
- After delivery and placental detachment, the highly vascular yet denuded uterus is widely exposed.
- Interference with the ability of the uterus to contract leads to uterine atony.
- Subsequently, the opened vessels at the site of placental attachment continue to bleed.
- Any condition that interferes with the ability of the uterus to contract can lead to uterine atony and, subsequently, to postpartum hemorrhage.

- Tearing of the uterine artery, such as with cervical lacerations or lacerations of the birth canal, can lead to hemorrhage.
- Abnormal placental implantation that leaves an area of separation between the placenta and decidua can lead to hemorrhage.

CAUSES

- Amnionitis
- Disseminated intravascular coagulation
- Incomplete placental separation
- Lacerations of the birth canal
- Rapid fetal descent
- Retained placental fragments
- Uterine atony
- Uterine inversion

ASSESSMENT FINDINGS

- Bleeding that can occur suddenly in large amounts or gradually as seeping or oozing of blood
- Frequent saturation of perineal pads
- In uterine atony, soft, relaxed uterus on palpation to the right or left of midline with distended bladder
- With retained placental fragments, soft noncontracting uterus on palpation and slow trickle, oozing, or frank hemorrhage
- With genital tract lacerations, continuous bright red vaginal bleeding and firm uterus
- With continuous or copious bleeding, signs and symptoms of hypovolemic shock:
  - Pallor
  - Decreased sensorium
  - Rapid, shallow respirations
  - Drop in urine output to less than 25 ml/hour
  - Rapid, thready peripheral pulses
  - Cold, clammy skin
  - Mean arterial pressure below 60 mm hg
  - Narrowing pulse pressure

ALERT Be alert for subtle changes in the patient's condition. Signs and symptoms of shock don't appear until hem-

orrhage is advanced because of the increased fluid and blood volumes of pregnancy.

TEST RESULTS

- Hemoglobin and hematocrit levels are decreased (a drop of 1 to 1.5 g/dl in hemoglobin level and approximately 2% to 4% drop in hematocrit from baseline).
- Urine specific gravity and osmolality (if shock ensues) are increased.
- Arterial blood pH and partial pressure of arterial oxygen are decreased; partial pressure of arterial carbon dioxide (if shock occurs) is increased.
- Platelet and fibrinogen levels, coagulation factors, and antithrombin III levels are decreased; prolonged clotting times are prolonged; and the D-dimer test (if DIC is the cause) is increased.

TREATMENT

▶ **COLLABORATION** *Caring for the patient with postpartum hemorrhage requires maximizing oxygenation, maintaining cardiopulmonary function and hemodynamic status, and reducing oxygen demand with rest and limitation of activity. The multidisciplinary approach might include involvement of intensive care unit personnel, a surgeon (for insertion of a central venous catheter, if indicated), and a neonatal specialist. Social services can helpful provide support for the patient, the neonate, and the family.*

- Correcting the underlying cause of the hemorrhage and instituting measures to control blood loss and minimize the extent of hypovolemic shock
- Emergency treatment: prompt and adequate blood and fluid replacement to restore intravascular volume and to raise blood pressure and maintain it above 60 mm Hg; rapid infusion of normal saline or lactated Ringer's solution and, possibly, blood products, albumin, or other plasma expanders to stabilize hemodynamic status
- If uterine atony is the cause of bleeding: intermittent uterine massage
  - Oxytocin if massage is ineffective or if the uterus can't be maintained in a contracted state
  - Possible bimanual massage if other measures prove ineffective

- Methylergonvine (Methergine), prostaglandins, or other agents to promote strong, sustained uterine contractions
- Arterial embolization if other therapies are ineffective
- Hysterectomy as a last resort
- Surgical repair for any lacerations
- Retained placental fragments removed by dilatation and curettage (D&C)
- Treatment of the underlying cause

KEY PATIENT OUTCOMES

The patient will:
- maintain adequate cardiac output
- maintain adequate fluid volume and urine output
- exhibit hemodynamic stability
- communicate feelings about her condition
- use available support systems to aid in coping
- remain free from complications associated with hemorrhage.

NURSING INTERVENTIONS

- Assess the patient's fundus and lochia frequently to detect changes; notify the physician if the fundus doesn't remain contracted or if lochia increases or becomes watery with a change in color.
- Perform fundal massage, as indicated.
- Remain with the patient, frequently reassessing the fundus.

ALERT *Keep in mind that the uterus may relax quickly after massage is completed, placing the patient at risk for continued hemorrhage and uterine atony.*
- Weigh perineal pads and monitor pad count.
- Turn the patient to the side and inspect the sheet beneath the buttocks for pooling of blood; if necessary, weigh disposable bed linen pads, adding this to the weight of the perineal pads to estimate blood loss.
- Inspect perineal area closely for oozing from any lacerations.
- Monitor vital signs frequently for changes, noting any trends such as a continuously rising pulse rate; report any changes immediately.
- Change patient's position slowly.
- Assess intake and output; report urine output of less than 30 ml/hour.

- Encourage the patient to void frequently.
- Anticipate the need for an indwelling urinary catheter if the patient can't void.

Interventions for hypovolemic shock

Be prepared to perform the following interventions if the patient develops signs and symptoms of hypovolemic shock.

- Begin an I.V. infusion with normal saline solution or lactated Ringer's solution delivered through a large-bore (14G to 18G) catheter; assist with insertion of a central venous line and pulmonary artery catheter for hemodynamic monitoring.
- Record blood pressure and pulse, respiratory, and peripheral pulse rates every 15 minutes until stable.
- Continuously monitor heart rhythm and neurologic status.
- Monitor cardiac output and central venous, right atrial, pulmonary artery, and pulmonary artery wedge pressures hourly or as ordered.

ALERT *During therapy, assess the patient's skin color and temperature, noting any changes. Cold, clammy skin may signal continuing peripheral vascular constriction, indicating progressive shock.*

- Watch for signs of impending coagulopathy, such as petechiae, bruising, bleeding, or oozing from gums or venipuncture sites.
- Anticipate the need for fluid replacement and blood component therapy, as ordered.
- Obtain arterial blood samples to measure arterial blood gas (ABG) levels.
- Administer oxygen by nasal cannula, face mask, or airway to ensure adequate tissue oxygenation, adjusting the oxygen flow rate as ABG results and pulse oximetry levels indicate.

ALERT *If the patient's systolic blood pressure drops below 80 mm Hg, increase the oxygen flow rate and notify the physician immediately. Systolic blood pressure below 80 mm Hg usually results in inadequate uterine perfusion with worsening of uterine atony, inadequate coronary artery blood flow, cardiac ischemia, arrhythmias, and further complications of low cardiac output. Expect to increase the infusion rate if the patient experiences a progressive drop in blood pressure accompanied by a* *thready pulse; this usually signals inadequate cardiac output from reduced intravascular volume.*

■ Obtain venous blood samples, as ordered, for a complete blood count, electrolyte levels, typing and crossmatching, and coagulation studies.

ALERT If the patient has received oxytocin I.V. for treatment of uterine atony, continue to assess the fundus closely. Oxytocin delivers immediate onset of action, but the duration of action is short, so the atony may reoccur.

■ If the health care provider orders prostaglandin therapy, be alert for possible adverse effects, such as nausea, diarrhea, tachycardia, and hypertension. Inform the patient about these effects.

■ Prepare the patient for possible treatments, such as bimanual massage, surgical repair of lacerations, or D&C, as indicated.

■ Provide emotional support to the patient; explain all events and treatments.

PATIENT TEACHING

Be sure to cover:

■ the disorder, diagnosis, and treatment

■ assessing lochia flow

■ measures to control bleeding

■ medications being administered

■ signs and symptoms of hemorrhage and the need to inform the health care provider.

Premature labor

DESCRIPTION

■ Onset of rhythmic uterine contractions that produce cervical changes after fetal viability but before fetal maturity

■ Usually occurs between 20 and 37 weeks' gestation

■ Fetal prognosis variable by birth weight and length of gestation

- Neonates who weigh less than 737 g and are less than 26 weeks' gestation have a survival rate of about 10%.

- Those who weigh 737 to 992 g and are between 27 and 28 weeks' gestation have a survival rate of more than 50%.

– Those who weigh 992 to 1,219 g and are more than 28 weeks' gestation have a 70% to 90% survival rate.
■ Increases risk of neonatal morbidity or mortality from excessive maturational deficiencies
■ Also called *preterm labor*

PATHOPHYSIOLOGY

■ Factors associated with the onset of labor include stretching of uterine muscle with subsequent release of prostaglandin, cervical pressure leading to release of oxytocin, change in ratio of estrogen to progesterone, placental age, rising fetal cortisol levels leading to reduced progesterone formation and increased prostaglandin formation, and fetal membrane production of prostaglandin.
■ The exact mechanism that triggers preterm labor is unclear.
■ Preterm labor is associated with dehydration, urinary tract infection, chorioamnionitis, uterine anomalies, and multiple gestation.

CAUSES

Maternal causes
■ Abdominal surgery or trauma
■ Cardiovascular and renal disease
■ Cervical insufficiency
■ Diabetes mellitus
■ Domestic violence
■ Gestational hypertension
■ Infection
■ Placental abnormalities
■ Premature rupture of membranes

Fetal causes
■ Fetal anomalies
■ Hydramnios
■ Infection
■ Multiple gestation

ASSESSMENT FINDINGS

- Onset of rhythmic uterine contractions
- Possible rupture of membranes, passage of the cervical mucus plug, and bloody discharge
- Typically 20 to 37 weeks' gestation
- Cervical effacement and dilation on vaginal examination
- Fetal fibronectin in cervicovaginal secretions

TEST RESULTS

- Ultrasonography shows fetal position and confirms the diagnosis.
- Urine and cervical cultures rule out the possibility of an infection.

TREATMENT

- Initial treatment to suppress preterm labor if tests show immature fetal lung development, cervical dilation of less than 4 cm, and the absence of factors that contraindicate continuation of pregnancy
- Typical treatments: bed rest, ensuring adequate hydration and, when necessary, drug therapy with a tocolytic
- Contraindications to tocolytics: gestation less than 20 weeks, cervical dilation greater than 4 cm, and cervical effacement greater than 50%
- Drugs used in preterm labor, including:
  - terbutaline (Brethine), a beta-adrenergic blocker and the most commonly used tocolytic
  - magnesium sulfate, typically the first drug used to halt contractions
  - indomethacin (Indocin), a prostaglandin synthesis inhibitor (typically not used after 32 weeks' gestation, to avoid premature closure of the ductus arteriosus)
  - nifedipine (Procardia), a calcium channel blocker (see *Drugs used in preterm labor*, page 68)
- For prevention in a patient with a history of premature labor, a purse-string suture (cerclage) inserted at 14 to 18 weeks' gestation for cervical insufficiency

DRUGS USED IN PRETERM LABOR

Terbutaline (Brethine)
- Beta-2 receptor stimulator that causes smooth-muscle relaxation
- Contraindicated in severe gestational hypertension and cardiac disease
- *Maternal adverse effects:* tachycardia, diarrhea, nervousness and tremors, nausea and vomiting, headache, hyperglycemia or hypoglycemia, hypokalemia, and pulmonary edema
- *Fetal adverse effects:* tachycardia, hypoxia, hypoglycemia, and hypocalcemia
- Antidote: propranolol (Inderal)

Magnesium sulfate
- Central nervous system (CNS) depressant that prevents reflux of calcium into the myometrial cells, thereby keeping the uterus relaxed
- Contraindicated in severe abdominal pain of unknown origin and oliguria
- *Maternal adverse effects:* drowsiness, flushing, warmth, nausea, headache, slurred speech, and blurred vision
- Toxicity: manifested by CNS depression in the mother, respirations fewer than 12 breaths/minute, hyporeflexia, oliguria, cardiac arrhythmias, and cardiac arrest
- *Fetal adverse effects:* hypotonia and bradycardia
- Antidote: calcium gluconate

Indomethacin (Indocin)
- Nonsteroidal anti-inflammatory that decreases production of prostaglandins, which are lipid compounds associated with the initiation of labor
- Contraindicated in GI bleeding, ulcers, rectal bleeding, and severe cardiovascular, renal, or hepatic disease (use cautiously)
- *Maternal adverse effects:* nausea, vomiting, and dyspepsia; additive CNS effects if given with magnesium sulfate
- *Fetal adverse effects:* premature closure of ductus arteriosus
- Antidote: none; discontinue drug

Nifedipine (Procardia)
- Calcium channel blocker that decreases the production of calcium, a substance associated with the initiation of labor
- Contraindicated in sick sinus syndrome and second- or third-degree atrioventricular heart block, and when systolic blood pressure is less than 90 mm Hg
- *Maternal adverse effects:* headache and flushing; additive CNS effects if given with magnesium sulfate
- *Fetal adverse effects:* minimal
- Antidote: none, discontinue drug

KEY PATIENT OUTCOMES

The patient will:
- report a decrease in contraction frequency and intensity, ultimately reporting cessation of contractions
- maintain intact membranes
- demonstrate a stable fetal heart rate and pattern
- remain free from complications associated with treatment
- continue through the pregnancy, giving birth to a viable neonate as close to term as possible.

NURSING INTERVENTIONS

- Closely observe the patient in preterm labor for signs of fetal or maternal distress, and provide comprehensive supportive care.
- Provide information about the hospital stay, potential for delivery of a premature neonate, and the possible need for neonatal intensive care.
- During attempts to suppress preterm labor, make sure the patient maintains bed rest, preferably in a lateral supine position; provide appropriate diversionary activities.
- Administer medications as ordered. (See *Administering terbutaline*, page 70.)
- Use sedatives and analgesics sparingly. Minimize the need for these agents by providing comfort measures, such as frequent repositioning and good perineal and back care.
- Monitor blood pressure, pulse rate, respirations, fetal heart rate, and uterine contraction pattern when administering a beta-adrenergic stimulant, a sedative, or an opioid. (Minimize adverse effects by keeping the patient in a side-lying position as much as possible to ensure adequate placental perfusion.)

ALERT *Monitor the status of contractions, notifying the physician if the patient experiences more than four contractions per hour, if the mother's pulse rises above 120 beats/ minute or her systolic blood pressure drops below 90 mm Hg, or if the fetus's heart rate rises above 180 beats/minute or drops below 110 beats/minute.*

- Administer fluids, as ordered.
- Frequently assess deep tendon reflexes when administering magnesium sulfate.

ADMINISTERING TERBUTALINE

I.V. terbutaline may be ordered for a woman in premature labor. When administering this drug, follow these steps:

- Obtain baseline maternal vital signs, fetal heart rate (FHR), and laboratory studies, including serum glucose and electrolyte levels and hematocrit.
- Institute external monitoring of uterine contractions and FHR.
- Prepare the drug with lactated Ringer's solution instead of dextrose and water to prevent additional glucose load and possible hyperglycemia.
- Administer as an I.V. piggyback infusion into a main I.V. solution so that the drug can be discontinued immediately if the patient experiences adverse reactions.
- Use microdrip tubing and an infusion pump to ensure an accurate flow rate.
- Expect to adjust the infusion flow rate every 10 minutes until contractions cease or adverse reactions become problematic.
- Monitor maternal vital signs every 15 minutes while the infusion rate is being increased and then every 30 minutes thereafter until contractions cease; monitor FHR every 15 to 30 minutes.
- Auscultate breath sounds for evidence of crackles or changes; monitor the patient for complaints of dyspnea and chest pain.
- Be alert for maternal pulse rate greater than 120 beats/minute, blood pressure less than 90/60 mm Hg, or persistent tachycardia or tachypnea, chest pain, dyspnea, or abnormal breath sounds because these could indicate developing pulmonary edema. Notify the physician immediately.
- Watch for fetal tachycardia or late or variable decelerations in FHR pattern because these could indicate uterine bleeding or fetal distress necessitating an emergency birth.
- Monitor intake and output closely, every hour during the infusion and then every 4 hours thereafter.
- Expect to continue the infusion for 12 to 24 hours after contractions have ceased and then to switch to oral therapy.
- Administer the first dose of oral therapy 30 minutes before discontinuing the I.V. infusion.
- Instruct the patient on how to take the oral therapy, continuing therapy until 37 weeks' gestation or until fetal lung maturity has been confirmed by amniocentesis; alternatively, if the patient is prescribed subcutaneous terbutaline therapy via a continuous pump, teach the patient how to use the pump.
- Teach the patient how to measure her pulse rate before each dose of oral terbutaline, or at the recommended times with subcutaneous therapy; instruct the patient to call the physician if her pulse rate exceeds 120 beats/minute or if she experiences palpitations or severe nervousness.

- Remember that a preterm neonate has a lower tolerance for the stress of labor and is much more likely to become hypoxic than a full-term neonate.
- If necessary, administer oxygen to the patient through a rebreather mask.
- Encourage the patient to lie on her left side or sit up during labor.
- Observe maternal and fetal responses to labor by continuous monitoring.
- Prevent maternal hyperventilation, using a rebreathing bag, as necessary.
- Provide emotional support and reassurance.
- Encourage use of nonpharmacologic pain management techniques.
- Avoid administering an analgesic when delivery is imminent.
- Monitor fetal and maternal responses to local and regional anesthetics.
- Monitor the neonate for signs of magnesium toxicity, including neuromuscular and respiratory depression.
- If labor is suppressed, begin discharge teaching with the patient and her family about tocolytic therapy at home; anticipate referral for home care follow-up.

PATIENT TEACHING

Be sure to cover:
- the disorder, diagnosis, and treatment
- signs and symptoms of premature labor and the need to notify the health care provider
- danger signs of labor that should be reported immediately
- medication therapy, including possible adverse effects
- importance of adherence to therapy and continued follow-up.

Premature rupture of membranes
DESCRIPTION

- Spontaneous break or tear in the amniotic sac before onset of regular contractions, resulting in progressive cervical dilation
- Premature rupture of membranes (PROM): membrane rupture 1 or more hours before the onset of labor

■ Preterm PROM: rupture of the membranes before the onset of labor in a preterm gestation

> **ALERT** *The mother is at risk for chorioamnionitis if the latent period (time between rupture of membranes and onset of labor) is longer than 24 hours. Signs include fetal tachycardia, maternal fever, foul-smelling amniotic fluid, and uterine tenderness. Development of chorioamnionitis can lead to sepsis and death. The risk of development increases exponentially after 18 hours of ruptured membranes without delivery.*

■ Risks: fetal infection, sepsis, and perinatal mortality (risks increase with every hour of ruptured membranes, every hour of labor, and every vaginal examination or other invasive procedure)

PATHOPHYSIOLOGY

■ The exact mechanism for premature rupture of membranes is unclear.

CAUSES

■ Exact cause unknown
■ Commonly accompanied by malpresentation and a contracted pelvis
■ Predisposing factors: poor nutrition and hygiene, lack of prenatal care, an incompetent cervix, increased intrauterine tension due to hydramnios or multiple pregnancies, defects in the amniotic membrane, and uterine, vaginal, and cervical infections (most commonly group B streptococcal, gonococcal, chlamydial, and anaerobic organisms)

ASSESSMENT FINDINGS

■ Typically, blood-tinged amniotic fluid containing vernix caseosa particles gushing or leaking from the vagina
■ Maternal fever, fetal tachycardia, and foul-smelling vaginal discharge (indicate infection)

TEST RESULTS

■ Alkaline pH of fluid collected from the posterior fornix turns the nitrazine paper deep blue.

- A smear of fluid, placed on a slide and allowed to dry, takes on a fern-like pattern because of the high sodium and protein content of the amniotic fluid.
- Transvaginal ultrasonography reveals a rupture or tear of the amniotic sac.

TREATMENT

- Depends on fetal age and the risk of infection
- In a term pregnancy, if spontaneous labor and vaginal delivery don't result within a relatively short time (usually within 24 hours after the membranes rupture): labor usually induced with oxytocin; if induction fails, cesarean delivery performed
- In a preterm pregnancy of less than 34 weeks: controversial management
- In a preterm pregnancy of 28 to 34 weeks: hospitalization and observation for signs of infection (such as maternal leukocytosis or fever, and fetal tachycardia) while awaiting fetal maturation
- If clinical status suggests infection: baseline cultures and sensitivity tests
- If these tests confirm infection: labor induced, followed by I.V. administration of an antibiotic and temperature monitoring every 2 hours
- Culture of gastric aspirate or a swabbing from the neonate's ear to determine the need for antibiotic therapy
- With delivery, resuscitation equipment readily available to treat neonatal distress

KEY PATIENT OUTCOMES

The patient will:
- maintain stable vital signs
- remain free from signs and symptoms of infection
- progress through the stages of labor without complications
- give birth to a viable neonate.

NURSING INTERVENTIONS

- Prepare the patient for a sterile vaginal examination.
- Before physically examining a patient who's suspected of having PROM, explain all diagnostic tests and answer any questions.
- During the examination, stay with the patient and offer reassurance.
- Assist with the examination, providing sterile gloves and sterile lubricating jelly.
- Don't use iodophor antiseptic solution when testing fluid with nitrazine paper.
- After the examination, provide proper perineal care.
- Maintain patient on bed rest; limit vaginal examinations.
- Send fluid specimens to the laboratory promptly.
- If the patient has streptococcal B infection, anticipate the need to administer a prophylactic antibiotic.
- Administer I.V. fluids as ordered.
- If labor starts, observe the mother's contractions and monitor her status; monitor vital signs every 2 hours.
- Watch for signs of maternal infection, such as fever, abdominal tenderness, and changes in amniotic fluid (including purulence or foul odor) and fetal tachycardia (which may precede maternal fever); report such signs immediately.
- Encourage the patient and her family to express their feelings and concerns about the neonate's health and survival.

PATIENT TEACHING

Be sure to cover:
- the disorder, diagnosis, and treatment
- signs and symptoms of PROM with the need to immediately report them to the health care provider
- tests and procedures used to confirm PROM
- avoidance of sexual intercourse, douching, or taking tub baths after the membranes rupture
- signs and symptoms of infection with the need to report immediately to the health care provider.

Life-threatening disorder

Prolapsed umbilical cord

DESCRIPTION

- Descent of the umbilical cord into the vagina before the presenting part (see *Umbilical cord prolapse*)
- May occur anytime after the membranes rupture (especially if the presenting part isn't fitted firmly in the cervix)

 ALERT *Umbilical cord prolapse is an emergency requiring prompt action to save the fetus; the cord may become compressed between the fetus and the maternal cervix or pelvis, thus compromising fetoplacental perfusion.*

PATHOPHYSIOLOGY

- A loop of the umbilical cord slips down in front of the fetal presenting part.
- The fetal presenting part compresses the cord at the pelvic brim.
- Compression leads to impaired perfusion.

FOCUS IN
UMBILICAL CORD PROLAPSE

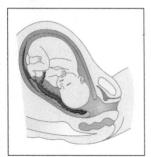

Umbilical cord prolapse with the cord remaining within the uterus

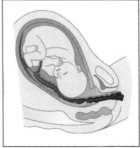

Umbilical cord prolapse with the cord appearing at the perineal area

- Prolapse of the cord to the outside leads to drying, with subsequent atrophy of the umbilical vessels or cord developing vasospasm, due to change in temperature or manual handling.

CAUSES

- Cephalopelvic disproportion preventing firm engagement
- Factors interfering with fetal descent
- Fetal presentation other than cephalic
- Hydramnios
- Intrauterine tumors preventing the presenting part from engaging
- Multiple gestation
- Placenta previa
- Premature rupture of membranes
- Small or preterm fetus

ASSESSMENT FINDINGS

- Cord possibly palpable at the perineum during vaginal examination or visible at the vulva
- Fetal heart rate (FHR) showing variable or prolonged decelerations

TEST RESULTS

- Ultrasonography confirms a prolapse.

TREATMENT

ALERT Measures to relieve pressure on the cord are initiated immediately. The patient is placed in the Trendelenburg (if cord isn't palpated in posterior cervical area) or knee-chest position (if evidence demonstrates uterus hasn't ruptured) to cause the fetal presenting part to fall back from the cord. Or, a sterile gloved hand may be inserted into the vagina to elevate the fetal head up and off the cord.

- Oxygen, usually
- Continuous FHR monitoring (if not already in place), with frequent observations for decelerations

- Saline-soaked sterile dressings over any exposed portion of the cord
- Vaginal delivery if the patient's cervix is fully dilated; cesarean delivery if cervical dilation is incomplete

KEY PATIENT OUTCOMES

The patient will:

- maintain stable vital signs
- remain free from complications
- demonstrate absence of fetal distress
- verbalize fears and concerns
- use effective coping strategies
- give birth to a viable neonate.

NURSING INTERVENTIONS

ALERT Always auscultate fetal heart sounds immediately after rupture of the membranes occurring either sponta-neously or by amniotomy.

- Assist with measures to relieve cord compression.
- Administer oxygen at 10 L/minute by face mask as ordered.
- Anticipate the use of a tocolytic.
- Monitor uterine contractions and FHR patterns closely; notify the physician of any variable decelerations.
- Cover any exposed areas of the cord with sterile saline-soaked dressings as ordered.
- Prepare the patient for delivery.
- Explain to the patient and her family what's happening and any treatments and procedures.
- Offer emotional support.

PATIENT TEACHING

Be sure to cover:

- the disorder, diagnosis, and treatment
- procedures and treatments being done
- signs and symptoms of fetal distress
- preparation for cesarean delivery, if indicated.

Sexually transmitted infections

DESCRIPTION

- Spread through sexual contact with an infected partner
- Increase the risk of complications in pregnancy (see *Selected STIs and pregnancy*, pages 80 to 83)
- Possible maternal complications: preterm labor chorioamnionitis, premature rupture of membranes, and endometritis after cesarean birth
- Possible fetal and neonatal complications: preterm birth, sepsis, and congenital infection

PATHOPHYSIOLOGY

- An organism invades the body.
- The resulting infection places the patient, the fetus or neonate at risk for complications.

CAUSES

- Bacteria such as *Chlamydia, Gonorrhea*
- Fungi such as *Candidiasis*
- Parasites such as pediculosis
- Protozoa such as *Trichomonas*
- Viruses such as human papilloma virus, human immunodeficiency virus

ASSESSMENT FINDINGS

- Typically, vaginal discharge or lesion
- Vulvar or vaginal irritation such as an itching or burning sensation

TEST RESULTS

- A culture of secretions is positive for organism.
- Organism is evident in blood.

TREATMENT

▶ **COLLABORATION** *Caring for the pregnant patient with a sexually transmitted infection (STI) requires a multidisciplinary approach. Infection control personnel may be required to help reduce the risk of transmission. Social services can assist in community referrals and support for follow-up.*

■ Pharmacologic therapy with antifungal, antimicrobial, or antiviral
■ Safer sex practices
■ Treatment of partner

KEY PATIENT OUTCOMES

The patient will:
■ verbalize understanding of STI and its possible effects on pregnancy
■ demonstrate appropriate infection control measures
■ exhibit improvement or healing of STI-related lesions
■ state relief of pain or discomfort
■ practice safe sex
■ remain free from signs and symptoms of infection
■ give birth to a term neonate free from infection.

NURSING INTERVENTIONS

■ Explain the mode of transmission of the STI, and educate the patient about measures to reduce the risk of transmission.
■ Administer drug therapy as ordered.
■ Instruct the patient in medication regimens as appropriate.
■ Stress the importance of completing the entire course of drug therapy.
■ Urge the patient to refrain from sexual intercourse until the active infection is completely gone.
■ Instruct the patient to inform any partners of the infection so that treatment can be initiated, thus preventing the risk of reinfection.
■ Provide comfort measures for the patient.
■ Instruct the patient to keep the vulvar area clean and dry.
■ Advise the patient to avoid using strong soaps, creams, or ointments unless prescribed.
■ Suggest the use of cool or tepid sitz baths to relieve itching.

(Text continues on page 84.)

SELECTED STIs AND PREGNANCY

This chart lists several sexually transmitted infections (STIs), their causative
organisms, assessment findings, and appropriate treatment for pregnant patients.

STI	Causative organism	Assessment findings
Chlamydia	*Chlamydia trachomatis*	■ Commonly produces no symptoms; suspicion raised if partner treated for nongonococcal urethritis ■ Heavy, gray-white vaginal discharge ■ Painful urination ■ Positive vaginal culture using special chlamydial test kit
Condyloma acuminata	Human papillomavirus	■ Discrete papillary structures that spread, enlarge, and coalesce to form large lesions; increasing in size during pregnancy ■ Possible secondary ulceration and infection with foul odor
Genital herpes	Herpes simplex virus, type 2	■ Painful, small vesicles with erythematous base on vulva or vagina rupturing within 1 to 7 days to form ulcers ■ Low-grade fever ■ Dyspareunia ■ Positive viral culture of vesicular fluid ■ Positive enzyme-linked immunosorbent assay
Gonorrhea	*Neisseria gonorrhoeae*	■ May not produce symptoms ■ Yellow-green vaginal discharge ■ Male partner who experiences severe pain on urination and purulent yellow penile discharge ■ Positive culture of vaginal, rectal, or urethral secretions

Treatment	Special considerations
■ Amoxicillin (Amoxil)	■ Screening for infection at first prenatal visit because it's one of the most common types of vaginal infection seen during pregnancy ■ Repeated screening in the third trimester if the woman has multiple sexual partners ■ Doxycycline (Vibramycin) — drug of choice for treatment if the woman isn't pregnant — contraindicated during pregnancy because of its association with fetal long bone deformities ■ Concomitant testing for gonorrhea because of the high incidence of concurrent infection ■ Possible premature rupture of membranes (PROM), preterm labor, and endometritis in the postpartum period resulting from infection ■ Possible development of conjunctivitis or pneumonia in neonate born to mother with infection present in the vagina
■ Topical application of trichloroacetic acid or bichloroacetic acid to lesions ■ Lesion removal with laser therapy, cryocautery, or knife excision	■ Serious infections associated with the development of cervical cancer later in life ■ Lesions left in place during pregnancy unless bothersome and removed during the postpartum period
■ Acyclovir (Zovirax) orally or in ointment form	■ Reduction or suppression of symptoms, shedding, or recurrent episodes only with drug therapy; not a cure for infection ■ Abstinence urged until vesicles completely heal ■ Primary infection transmission possible across the placenta, resulting in congenital infection in the neonate ■ Transmission to neonate possible if active lesions are present in the vagina or on the vulva at birth, which can be fatal ■ Cesarean delivery recommended if patient has active lesions
■ Cefixime (Suprax) as a one-time I.M. injection	■ Associated with spontaneous miscarriage, preterm birth, and endometritis in the postpartum period ■ Treatment of sexual partners required to prevent reinfection ■ Major cause of pelvic infectious disease and infertility ■ Severe eye infection leading to blindness in the neonate (ophthalmia neonatorum) if infection present at birth

(continued)

SELECTED STIs AND PREGNANCY (continued)

STI	Causative organism	Assessment findings
Group B streptococci infection	Spirochete	■ Usually produces no symptoms
Syphilis	*Treponema pallidum*	■ Painless ulcer on vulva or vagina (primary syphilis) ■ Hepatic and splenic enlargement, headache, anorexia, and maculopapular rash on the palms of the hands and soles of the feet (secondary syphilis; occurring about 2 months after initial infection) ■ Cardiac, vascular, and central nervous system changes (tertiary syphilis; occurring after an undetermined latent phase) ■ Positive Venereal Disease Research Laboratory serum test; confirmed with positive rapid plasma reagin and fluorescent treponemal antibody absorption tests ■ Dark-field microscopy positive for spirochete
Trichomoniasis	Single-cell protozoan infection	■ Yellow-gray, frothy, odorous vaginal discharge ■ Vulvar itching, edema, and redness ■ Vaginal secretions on a wet slide treated with potassium hydroxide positive for organism
Vaginosis, bacterial	*Gardnerella vaginalis* infection (most commonly)	■ Thin, gray vaginal discharge with a fishlike odor ■ Intense pruritus ■ Wet mount slide positive for clue cells (epithelial cells with numerous bacilli clinging to the cells' surface)

Treatment	Special considerations
■ Broad-spectrum penicillin such as ampicillin	■ Occurs in as many as 15% to 35% of pregnant women ■ May lead to urinary tract infection, intra-amniotic infection leading to preterm birth, and postpartum endometritis ■ Screening for all pregnant women recommended by the Centers for Disease Control and Prevention at 35 to 38 weeks' gestation
■ Penicillin G benzathine (Bicillin L-A) I.M. (single dose)	■ Possible transmission across placenta after approximately 18 weeks' gestation, leading to spontaneous miscarriage, preterm labor, stillbirth, or congenital anomalies in the neonate ■ Standard screening for syphilis at the first prenatal visit, screening at 36 weeks' gestation for women with multiple partners, and possible rescreening at beginning of labor, with neonates tested for congenital syphilis using a sample of cord blood ■ Jarisch-Herxheimer reaction (sudden hypotension, fever, tachycardia, and muscle aches) after medication administration, lasting for about 24 hours, and then fading because spirochetes are destroyed
■ Topical clotrimazole (Gyne-Lotrimin) instead of metronidazole (Flagyl) because of its possible teratogenic effects if used during the first trimester of pregnancy	■ Possibly associated with preterm labor, PROM, and postcesarean infection ■ Treatment of partner required, even if asymptomatic
■ Topical vaginal metronidazole after the first trimester, usually late in pregnancy	■ Rapid growth and multiplication of organisms, replacing the normal lactobacilli organisms that are found in the healthy woman's vagina ■ Treatment goal of reestablishing the normal balance of vaginal flora ■ Untreated infections associated with amniotic fluid infections and, possibly, preterm labor and PROM

- Encourage the patient to wear cotton underwear and to avoid tight-fighting clothing as much as possible.
- Instruct the patient in safer sex practices, including the use of condoms and spermicides such as nonoxynol 9.
- Emphasize the importance of early diagnosis and treatment.
- Encourage follow-up.

PATIENT TEACHING

Be sure to cover:
- the disorder, diagnosis, and treatment
- need to inform sexual partners of infection so they can seek treatment
- infection control measures
- avoidance of sexual contact until advised by the health care provider
- importance of compliance with prescribed therapy and follow-up.

Spontaneous abortion
DESCRIPTION

- Expelled products of conception from the uterus before fetal viability
- Classified according to types (see *Types of spontaneous abortion*)
- Occurs in about 10% to 20% of first pregnancies and 15% of all pregnancies
- Typically occurs in first trimester (75%)
- Possible complications: infection, hemorrhage, anemia, coagulation defects, disseminated intravascular coagulation, and psychological issues of loss and failure
- Also called *miscarriage*

PATHOPHYSIOLOGY

- Spontaneous abortion may result from fetal, placental, or maternal factors.
- Defective embryologic development, faulty implantation of fertilized ovum, and failure of the endometrium to accept the fertilized ovum are common factors leading to abortion between 9 and 12 weeks' gestation.
- Placental factors, including inadequate hormone production, premature separation of a normally implanted placenta, and abnormal pla-

TYPES OF SPONTANEOUS ABORTION

Depending on clinical findings, a spontaneous abortion (miscarriage) may be threatened or inevitable, incomplete or complete, or missed, habitual, or septic. Here's how the seven types compare.

Threatened abortion

Bloody vaginal discharge occurs during the first half of pregnancy. About 20% of pregnant women have vaginal spotting or actual bleeding early in pregnancy; of these, about 50% abort.

Inevitable abortion

The membranes rupture and the cervix dilates. As labor continues, the uterus expels the products of conception.

Incomplete abortion

The uterus retains part or all of the placenta. Before 10 weeks' gestation, the fetus and placenta usually are expelled together; after the 10th week, they're expelled separately. Because part of the placenta may adhere to the uterine wall, bleeding continues. Hemorrhage is possible because the uterus doesn't contract and seal the large vessels that fed the placenta.

Complete abortion

The uterus passes all the products of conception. Minimal bleeding usually accompanies complete abortion because the uterus contracts and compresses the maternal blood vessels that fed the placenta.

Missed abortion

The uterus retains the products of conception for 2 months or more after the death of the fetus. Uterine growth ceases; uterine size may even seem to decrease. Prolonged retention of the dead products of conception may cause coagulation defects such as disseminated intravascular coagulation.

Habitual abortion

Spontaneous loss of three or more consecutive pregnancies constitutes habitual abortion.

Septic abortion

Infection accompanies abortion. This may occur with spontaneous abortion but usually results from an illegal abortion or from the presence of an intrauterine device.

cental implantation or function, usually lead to abortion around 14 weeks' gestation (when the placenta takes over the hormone production necessary to maintain pregnancy).

■ Maternal factors, including use of a teratogenic drug, malnutrition, and abnormalities of the reproductive organs (weakened cervix), usually lead to abortion between 11 and 19 weeks' gestation.

CAUSES

■ Abnormalities of the reproductive organs
■ Blood group incompatibility and Rh isoimmunization
■ Cervical insufficiency
■ Diabetes mellitus
■ Environmental toxins
■ Fetal factors
■ Lowered estriol secretion
■ Maternal infection
■ Placental factors
■ Recreational drug use
■ Severe malnutrition
■ Surgery that necessitates manipulation of the pelvic organs
■ Thyroid gland dysfunction
■ Trauma

ASSESSMENT FINDINGS

■ Pink discharge for several days or scant brown discharge for several weeks before onset of cramps and increased vaginal bleeding
■ Cramps that appear for a few hours, intensify, then occur more frequently
■ Vaginal bleeding
■ Cervical dilation
■ Passage of nonviable products of conception
■ Continued cramps and bleeding if any uterine contents remain (cramps and bleeding may subside if entire contents expelled)

TEST RESULTS

■ Levels of serum human chorionic gonadotropin are decreased.
■ Products of conception as shown by cytologic analysis are evident.

- Levels of serum hemoglobin and hematocrit due to blood loss are decreased.
- Ultrasonography reveals the absence of fetal heart tones or an empty amniotic sac.

TREATMENT

- Accurate evaluation of uterine contents before planning treatment
- Progression of spontaneous abortion unavoidable, except in those cases caused by cervical insufficiency
- Hospitalization to control severe hemorrhage
- Possible bed rest
- Transfusion with packed red blood cells or whole blood for severe bleeding
- I.V. oxytocin to stimulate uterine contractions
- Dilatation and curettage or dilatation and evacuation if remnants remain in the uterus
- Possible surgical reinforcement of the cervix (cerclage) to prevent abortion
- For an Rh-negative patient with a negative indirect Coombs' test result: $Rh_o(D)$ immune globulin

KEY PATIENT OUTCOMES

The patient will:

- exhibit no signs and symptoms of infection
- communicate feelings about the current situation
- use available support systems, such as family and friends, to aid in coping.

NURSING INTERVENTIONS

- Don't allow bathroom privileges because the patient may expel uterine contents without knowing it.
- Inspect bedpan contents carefully for intrauterine material.
- Monitor vital signs and intake and output.
- Assess amount, color, and odor of vaginal bleeding; perform pad count, and save all sanitary pads for evaluation.
- Administer prescribed drugs.
- Provide perineal care.
- Provide emotional support and counseling.

- Encourage expression of feelings.
- Help the patient develop effective coping strategies. Refer to professional counseling, if indicated.

PATIENT TEACHING

Be sure to cover:
- the disorder, diagnosis, and treatment
- vaginal bleeding or spotting
- need to report bleeding that lasts longer than 8 to 10 days, excessive bleeding, or bright red blood
- signs of infection, such as fever and foul-smelling vaginal discharge
- gradual resumption of daily activities
- schedule for returning to work (normally within 1 to 4 weeks)
- abstinence from intercourse for 1 to 2 weeks
- prevention of spontaneous abortion
- contraceptive information
- need to avoid use of tampons for 1 to 2 weeks
- need for follow-up examination.

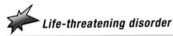 *Life-threatening disorder*

Uterine rupture

DESCRIPTION

- Occurs in about 1 in 1,500 births (rare)
- Factors affecting fetal viability: extent of the rupture and time lapse between rupture and cesarean deliver
- Factors affecting maternal prognosis: extent of the rupture and blood loss

PATHOPHYSIOLOGY

- Excessive strain to the uterus can cause a uterine rupture.
- A pathologic retraction ring may precede a uterine rupture. (See *Understanding a pathologic retraction ring*.)
- Involvement of the endometrium, myometrium, and peritoneum may indicate a complete rupture.
- No involvement of the peritoneum may indicate an incomplete rupture.

CAUSES

- Hysterotomy repair
- Prolonged labor, faulty presentation, multiple gestation, oxytocin use, obstructed labor, and traumatic maneuvers using forceps or traction
- Uterine anomalies
- Vertical scar as a result of previous cesarean delivery

ASSESSMENT FINDINGS

- Indentation appearing across the abdomen over the uterus (pathologic retraction ring)
- Strong uterine contractions without any cervical dilation

Complete uterine rupture

- Sudden, severe pain during a strong labor contraction
- Report of a tearing sensation
- Cessation of uterine contractions
- Hemorrhage

FOCUS IN
UNDERSTANDING A PATHOLOGIC RETRACTION RING

A pathologic retraction ring, also called *Bandl's ring*, is the most common type of constriction ring responsible for dysfunctional labor. It's a key warning sign of impending uterine rupture.

A pathologic retraction ring appears as a horizontal indentation across the abdomen, usually during the second stage of labor (see arrow in the illustration). The myometrium above the ring is considerably thicker than it is below the ring. When present, the ring prevents further passage of the fetus, holding the fetus in place at the point of the retraction. The placenta is also held at that point.

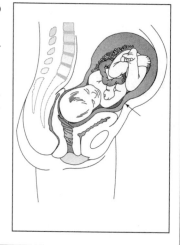

- Signs of shock, including falling blood pressure, cold and clammy skin, respiratory distress, and rapid, weak pulse
- Change in abdominal contour with two distinct swellings indicating retracted uterus and an extrauterine fetus
- Absence of fetal heart sounds

Incomplete uterine rupture

- Localized tenderness and persistent ache over lower uterine segment
- Gradual onset of fetal bradycardia, absence of fetal heart sounds, absence of contractions, and changes in maternal vital signs

TEST RESULTS

- The extent of rupture and blood loss affects test results.
- Arterial blood gas levels may reveal hypoxemia, decreased blood pH, and decreased partial pressure of arterial oxygen; partial pressure of arterial carbon dioxide may be increased.
- Urine specific gravity and urine osmolarity may be increased.

TREATMENT

> **COLLABORATION** *The patient with uterine rupture requires emergency management to promptly and adequately replace blood and fluids to restore intravascular volume and raise blood pressure. Respiratory therapists may be needed if the patient requires intubation and mechanical ventilation. A surgeon may be involved if a laparotomy is necessary after vaginal delivery. Renal specialists and dialysis may be required if the patient experiences renal failure. A neurologist or neurosurgeon may be needed if the patient continues to exhibit decreased mentation despite adequate resuscitation.*

> **ALERT** *At the end of pregnancy, the uterus is a highly vascular organ, making uterine rupture an immediate emergency situation, comparable to a splenic or hepatic rupture.*

- Emergency fluid replacement and I.V. oxytocin administration to contract the uterus and minimize bleeding
- Cesarean delivery, if possible

- Manual removal of the placenta under general anesthesia (with placental-stage pathologic retraction rings)
- Laparotomy after vaginal delivery to control bleeding and repair the rupture, if indicated; possible hysterectomy or tubal ligation

KEY PATIENT OUTCOMES

The patient will:
- maintain stable vital signs and cardiac output
- maintain adequate fluid balance
- remain free from complications
- express feelings related to the seriousness of her condition
- demonstrate appropriate coping mechanisms
- give birth to a viable neonate.

NURSING INTERVENTIONS

- Administer emergency fluid replacement therapy as ordered.
- Anticipate the use of I.V. oxytocin.
- Prepare the patient for a possible laparotomy.
- Inform the patient's family about her condition and prognosis, the extent of surgery, and the outcome for the fetus.
- Offer emotional support.

PATIENT TEACHING

Be sure to cover:
- the disorder, diagnosis, and treatment
- all procedures and equipment and their purpose
- preoperative and postoperative teaching
- inadvisability of another pregnancy (unless rupture occurred in the inactive lower segment).

NEONATAL

 Life-threatening disorder

Apnea

DESCRIPTION

- Cessation of breathing for 20 seconds, or less than 20 seconds if accompanied by color changes and bradycardia
- Commonly seen in preterm neonates and neonates with secondary stress, such as those with infection, hyperbilirubinemia, hypoglycemia, or hypothermia

PATHOPHYSIOLOGY

- The respiratory control centers located in the brain are immature.
- Additionally, the amount of surfactant may be insufficient.

CAUSES

- Acidosis
- Anemia
- Hypocalcemia
- Hypoglycemia or hyperglycemia
- Hypothermia or hyperthermia
- Immaturity
- Sepsis
- Upper airway obstruction

ASSESSMENT FINDINGS

- Breathing stops for more than 20 seconds
- Bradycardia
- Early cyanosis
- Oxygen saturation level less than 90%

TEST RESULTS

- Arterial blood gas (ABG) analysis reveals decreased partial pressure of oxygen and pH with increased partial pressure of carbon dioxide.

- Chest X-ray identifies pneumonia, fluid in the lungs, or structural abnormalities that might interfere with respirations.
- Blood glucose levels reveal hypoglycemia or hyperglycemia.
- Blood cultures rule out an infectious process.

TREATMENT

▶ **COLLABORATION** *Pulmonary specialists may be needed to assist with and treat the neonate's respiratory problems. If an infection is the cause of the neonate's apnea, an infectious disease specialist may become involved. An endocrinologist may be consulted to assist with controlling blood glucose level. Also, nutritional support may be needed to ensure adequate calorie intake for weight gain to support metabolic needs and foster growth and development. Respiratory therapy can help with respiratory support and monitoring, including apnea monitoring. Social services would be important to assist with coping and ease the transition to home. Referrals for home health care nursing and home apnea monitoring equipment may also be required.*

- Respiratory support
- Tactile stimulation
- Correction of underlying cause
- Gentle handling
- Evaluation of ABG and oxygen saturation levels
- Suctioning
- Home apnea monitoring
- Use of caffeine or administration of medications such as theophylline (Slo-Phyllin)

KEY PATIENT OUTCOMES

The patient will:
- maintain adequate ventilation
- maintain a patent airway
- demonstrate spontaneous breathing efforts
- maintain a stable body temperature.

NURSING INTERVENTIONS

- Assess respiratory status closely and frequently, including after feeding.

TEACHING ABOUT HOME APNEA MONITORING

Be sure to include the following topics in your teaching plan for the parents of a neonate receiving home apnea monitoring:
- rationale for use
- signs and symptoms of apnea
- equipment and procedure for use
- frequency and duration of use
- signs and symptoms requiring notification of the health care provider
- measures to stimulate respirations
- cardiopulmonary resuscitation technique
- follow-up care.

- Use an apnea monitor to help detect episodes; have emergency resuscitation equipment readily available.
- If apnea is noted, gently startle the neonate by flicking his sole.
- Anticipate the need for ventilatory support if the neonate experiences frequent apneic episodes, if the episodes are difficult to correct, or if oxygen saturation is less than 94%.
- Maintain a neutral thermal environment.
- Handle the neonate gently.
- Avoid measuring the neonate's temperature rectally, which causes vagal stimulation and, subsequently, bradycardia and apnea.

PATIENT TEACHING

Be sure to cover with the parents:
- the disorder, diagnosis, and treatment
- procedures, including respiratory support measures
- measures to stimulate the neonate
- home apnea monitoring, if ordered. (See *Teaching about home apnea monitoring.*)

Drug exposure
DESCRIPTION

- Results from maternal drug use during pregnancy
- Associated risks: urogenital malformations, cerebrovascular complica-

tions, low birth weight, decreased head circumference, respiratory problems, drug withdrawal, and death
- Neonatal abstinence syndrome (NAS): a constellation of neurologic and physical behaviors exhibited by drug-exposed neonates

PATHOPHYSIOLOGY

- Neonatal drug addiction results from intrauterine exposure.
- The drug acts as a teratogen, causing abnormalities in embryonic or fetal development.

CAUSES

- Intrauterine exposure to drugs, including:
    - Amphetamines
    - Cocaine
    - Heroin
    - Marijuana
    - Methadone
    - Opiates

ASSESSMENT FINDINGS

- High-pitched cry
- Jitteriness
- Tremors
- Irritability
- Poor feeding habits
- Hyperactive Moro reflex
- Increased deep tendon reflexes
- Frequent sneezing and yawning
- Poor sleeping pattern
- Diarrhea
- Vigorous sucking on hands
- Low birth weight or small for gestational age
- Signs and symptoms of withdrawal; dependent on the length of maternal addiction, the drug ingested, and the time of last ingestion before delivery (usually within 24 to 48 hours of delivery) (see *Signs and symptoms of opiate withdrawal*, page 96)

SIGNS AND SYMPTOMS OF OPIATE WITHDRAWAL

Central nervous system signs and symptoms	GI signs and symptoms	Autonomic signs and symptoms
■ Seizures ■ Tremors ■ Irritability ■ Increased wakefulness ■ High-pitched cry ■ Increased muscle tone ■ Increased deep tendon reflexes ■ Increased Moro reflex ■ Increased yawning ■ Increased sneezing ■ Rapid changes in mood ■ Hypersensitivity to noise and external stimuli	■ Poor feeding ■ Uncoordinated and constant sucking ■ Vomiting ■ Diarrhea ■ Dehydration ■ Poor weight gain	■ Increased sweating ■ Nasal stuffiness ■ Fever ■ Mottling ■ Temperature instability ■ Increased respiratory rate ■ Increased heart rate

TEST RESULTS

- Toxicology screen of urine or meconium is positive for drug use.
- Cultures are negative for an infectious agent.

TREATMENT

- Tight swaddling for comfort
- Quiet, dark environment to decrease environmental stimuli
- Pacifier to meet sucking needs (heroin withdrawal)
- Gavage feeding for poor sucking reflex (methadone withdrawal)
- Maintenance of fluid and electrolyte balance
- Avoidance of breast-feeding
- Assessment for jaundice (methadone withdrawal)
- Medication—such as opium (Paregoric), phenobarbital, chlorpro-mazine (Thorazine), or diazepam (Valium) to treat wthdrawal manifestations
- Promotion of maternal-infant bonding
- Evaluation for referral to child protective services, if warranted

KEY PATIENT OUTCOMES

The patient will:

- maintain a patent airway and adequate ventilation
- remain free from injury
- exhibit comfort
- ingest adequate nutrition
- demonstrate appropriate weight gain
- demonstrate positive bonding behaviors.

NURSING INTERVENTIONS

- Provide supportive care.
- Maintain a patent airway; have resuscitative equipment readily available.
- Elevate the neonate's head during feeding; offer a pacifier if the neonate demonstrates vigorous sucking (common in neonates of heroin-addicted mothers).
- Provide small, frequent feedings, positioning the nipple to ensure effective sucking.
- Monitor weight daily.
- Assess intake and output frequently, and monitor fluid and electrolyte balance.
- Administer supplemental fluids as ordered.
- Assess the neonate for signs and symptoms of respiratory distress, and report them immediately if present.
- Assess breath sounds frequently for changes.
- Administer supplemental oxygen, as ordered, and assist with ventilatory support.
- Monitor arterial blood gas values and transcutaneous oxygen levels.
- Cluster care and allow for adequate rest.
- Firmly swaddle the neonate.
- Protect the neonate from injury during seizures.
- Maintain skin integrity; provide meticulous skin care, and frequently change the neonate's position.

PATIENT TEACHING

Be sure to cover with the parents:
- the disorder, diagnosis, and treatment
- nutrition and feeding
- comfort measures
- withdrawal signs and symptoms
- methods to promote bonding and attachment.

Fetal alcohol syndrome

DESCRIPTION

- A cluster of birth defects resulting from in utero exposure to alcohol (see *Terminology associated with FAS*)
- Includes at least one abnormality in each of the following categories: growth retardation, central nervous system (CNS) abnormalities, and facial malformations
- Commonly found in neonates of women who ingested varying amounts of alcohol during pregnancy
- Can develop in the first 3 to 8 weeks of pregnancy, before a patient even knows she's pregnant
- Risks:
  - Occurs with even moderate alcohol consumption (1 to 2 oz [30 to 59 ml] of alcohol daily)
  - Increases proportionally with increased daily alcohol intake

PATHOPHYSIOLOGY

- Alcohol is a teratogenic substance that's particularly dangerous during critical periods of organogenesis.
- Alcohol interferes with the passage of amino acids across the placental barrier.
- Alcohol consumed by the pregnant patient crosses through the placenta and enters the blood supply of the fetus.
- Variables that affect the extent of damage caused to the fetus by alcohol include the amount of alcohol consumed, timing of consumption, and pattern of alcohol use.

CAUSES

- Intrauterine exposure to alcohol ingested by the mother during pregnancy

ASSESSMENT FINDINGS

- Prenatal and postnatal growth retardation
- Characteristic findings within the first 24 hours of life:
  - Difficulty establishing respirations

TERMINOLOGY ASSOCIATED WITH FAS

Fetal alcohol syndrome (FAS) is characterized by physical and mental disorders apparent at birth and problematic throughout the child's life. A distinctive pattern of three specific findings characterizes FAS: growth restriction (prenatal and postnatal); craniofacial structural anomalies, and central nervous system dysfunction. However, because effects other than those typically associated with FAS also occur, additional terminology has been developed to address these concerns.

■ *Fetal alcohol effects (FAE)* is used to describe children with a variety of problems thought to be associated with alcohol consumption by the mother during pregnancy. These problems may include low birth weight, developmental delays, and hyperactivity.

■ *Alcohol-related birth defects (ARBD)* is used to describe neonates with some but not all of the symptoms of FAS.

■ *Alcohol-related neurologic defects (ARND)* is used to describe neonates with neurologic symptoms associated with FAS, such as cognitive difficulties, hyperactivity problems, and mental impairments.

When the effects of prenatal exposure to alcohol are viewed on a continuum, FAS is considered severe.

– Irritability
– Lethargy
– Seizure activity
– Tremulousness
– Opisthotonos
– Poor sucking reflex
– Abdominal distention

■ Facial anomalies, such as microcephaly, micro-ophthalmia, maxillary hypoplasia, and short palpebral fissures (see *Common facial characteristics of neonates with FAS*, page 100)

■ CNS dysfunction, including decreased IQ, developmental delays, and neurologic abnormalities, such as decreased muscle tone, poor coordination, and a small brain

TEST RESULTS

■ No specific test confirms the diagnosis.

■ Radiography may reveal associated renal or cardiac defects.

COMMON FACIAL CHARACTERISTICS OF NEONATES WITH FAS

Eyes	■ Short palpebral fissures
	■ Strabismus
	■ Ptosis
	■ Myopia
Nose	■ Short
	■ Upturned
	■ Flat or absent groove above upper lip
Mouth	■ Thin upper lip
	■ Receding jaw

TREATMENT

- Prevention through public education
- Careful prenatal history and education
- Identification of women at risk, with referral to alcohol treatment centers, if necessary
- Prompt identification of neonates with FAS to ensure early intervention and appropriate referrals

KEY PATIENT OUTCOMES

The patient will:
- maintain a patent airway and adequate ventilation
- remain free from injury
- remain free from overstimulation
- ingest adequate nutrients to foster growth
- exhibit weight gain within acceptable parameters
- demonstrate bonding and attachment behaviors with the caregiver.

NURSING INTERVENTIONS

- Institute measures for prevention:
  - Increase public awareness about the dangers of alcohol consumption during pregnancy.
  - Ensure increased access to prenatal care.
  - Provide educational programs.

- Assist with screening women of reproductive age for alcohol problems.
- Use appropriate resources and strategies for decreasing alcohol use.
■ Closely assess any neonate born to a mother who has used alcohol.
■ Prevent and treat respiratory distress, including assessing breath sounds frequently, being alert for signs of distress, and suctioning as needed.
■ Encourage successful feeding; assist with developing measures to enhance the neonate's intake.
■ Monitor weight, and measure intake and output.
■ Promote parent-neonate attachment; encourage frequent visiting and rooming in, if possible, with physical contact between the parent and the neonate.
■ Provide emotional support and anticipatory guidance related to the neonate's condition.
■ Refer to social services to evaluate the home situation and to assess the neonate's home health needs, if indicated.

PATIENT TEACHING

Be sure to cover with the parents:
■ the disorder, diagnosis, and treatment
■ measures to facilitate bonding
■ nutritional needs and strategies
■ complications
■ danger signs and symptoms to report to the primary care provider
■ need for long-term follow-up.

 Life-threatening disorder

Hemolytic disease
DESCRIPTION

■ Hemolytic disease of the fetus and neonate
■ Stems from an incompatibility of fetal and maternal blood
■ Potential complications: fetal death in utero, severe anemia, heart failure, and kernicterus
■ Also called *hemolytic disease of the newborn, erythroblastosis fetalis*

PATHOPHYSIOLOGY

ABO incompatibility

- Each blood group has specific antigens on red blood cells (RBCs) and specific antibodies in the serum.
- The maternal immune system forms antibodies against fetal cells when blood groups differ.
- This can cause hemolytic disease even if fetal erythrocytes don't escape into the maternal circulation during pregnancy.

Rh incompatibility

- During her first pregnancy, an Rh-negative female becomes sensitized (during delivery or abortion) by exposure to Rh-positive fetal blood antigens inherited from the father. (See also "Isoimmunization," page 45.)
- A female may also become sensitized from receiving blood transfusions with alien Rh antigens, from inadequate doses of $Rh_0(D)$ (RhoGAM), or from failure to receive $Rh_0(D)$ after significant fetal-maternal leakage during abruptio placentae (premature detachment of the placenta).
- A subsequent pregnancy with an Rh-positive fetus provokes maternal production of agglutinating antibodies, which cross the placental barrier, attach to Rh-positive cells in the fetus, and cause hemolysis and anemia.
- To compensate, the fetal blood-forming organs step up the production of RBCs and erythroblasts (immature RBCs) appear in the fetal circulation.
- Extensive hemolysis releases more unconjugated bilirubin than the liver can conjugate and excrete, causing hyperbilirubinemia and hemolytic anemia.

CAUSES

- ABO incompatibility — frequently occurs during a first pregnancy; present in approximately 12% of pregnancies
- Rh isoimmunization (see *What happens in Rh isoimmunization*)
- Rh negativity — more common in Whites than in Blacks; rare in Asians
- Rh sensitization — 11 cases per 10,000 births

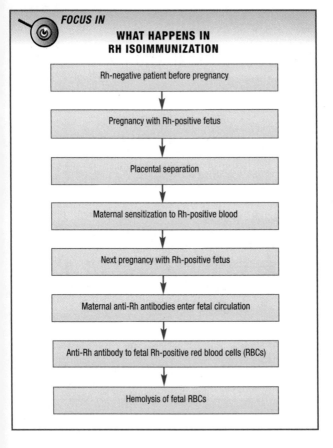

FOCUS IN

WHAT HAPPENS IN RH ISOIMMUNIZATION

Rh-negative patient before pregnancy

↓

Pregnancy with Rh-positive fetus

↓

Placental separation

↓

Maternal sensitization to Rh-positive blood

↓

Next pregnancy with Rh-positive fetus

↓

Maternal anti-Rh antibodies enter fetal circulation

↓

Anti-Rh antibody to fetal Rh-positive red blood cells (RBCs)

↓

Hemolysis of fetal RBCs

ASSESSMENT FINDINGS

- Mother Rh-positive, father Rh-negative, and antigen-antibody response developed during previous pregnancy
- History of blood transfusion in the mother
- Maternal history of erythroblastotic stillbirths, abortions, previously affected children, or previous anti-Rh titers
- Pallor
- Edema

- Petechiae
- Bile-stained umbilical cord
- Yellow- or meconium-stained amniotic fluid
- Mild to moderate hepatosplenomegaly
- Pulmonary crackles
- Heart murmur
- Jaundice

TEST RESULTS

- Paternal blood typing for ABO and Rh is necessary.
- Amniotic fluid analysis shows increased bilirubin and anti-Rh titers.
- Direct Coombs' test of umbilical cord blood measures RBC (Rh-positive) antibodies in the neonate (positive only when the mother is Rh negative and the fetus is Rh positive).
- Cord hemoglobin level in the neonate is less than 10 g, indicating severe disease.
- Many nucleated peripheral RBCs are present.
- Radiologic studies show edema and, in hydrops fetalis, the halo sign (edematous, elevated, subcutaneous fat layers) and the Buddha position (fetus's legs are crossed).

TREATMENT

- Phototherapy (exposure to ultraviolet light to reduce bilirubin levels)
- Intubation of neonate
- Removal of excess fluid
- Maintenance of body temperature
- Intrauterine-intraperitoneal transfusion (if amniotic fluid analysis suggests the fetus is severely affected and isn't mature enough to deliver)
- Exchange transfusion
- Albumin infusion
- Gamma globulin containing anti-Rh antibody ($Rh_o[D]$)
- Planned delivery (usually 2 to 4 weeks before term date, depending on maternal history, serologic test results, and amniocentesis)

KEY PATIENT OUTCOMES

The patient will:
- exhibit adequate ventilation

- remain hemodynamically stable
- maintain fluid balance within normal limits
- maintain normal temperature.

NURSING INTERVENTIONS

- Encourage expression of fears by the family concerning possible complications of treatment.
- Prepare the neonate for treatment procedures, such as phototherapy or exchange transfusion.
- Promote normal parental bonding.
- Administer $Rh_o(D)$ I.M. as ordered.
- Monitor cardiac rhythm and rate, airway and ventilation, and vital signs closely.
- Assist with transfusions, as ordered, and monitor for transfusion complications.
- Assess intake and output frequently.
- Encourage adherence to follow-up appointments.

PATIENT TEACHING

Be sure to cover with the parents:
- the disorder, diagnosis, and treatment
- medications, drug routes, and administration
- preventive measures for recurrence.

Hydrocephalus
DESCRIPTION

- A variety of conditions characterized by excess fluid within the cranial vault, subarachnoid space, or both
- Occurs because of interference with cerebrospinal fluid (CSF) flow caused by increased fluid production, obstruction within the ventricular system, or defective reabsorption of CSF
- Types:
  - Noncommunicating hydrocephalus: obstruction within the ventricular system (more common in children)
  - Communicating hydrocephalus: impaired absorption of CSF (more common in adults)

- Potential complications: mental retardation, impaired motor function, vision loss, infection and malnutrition, and death (from increased intracranial pressure [ICP])

PATHOPHYSIOLOGY

- The obstruction of CSF flow associated with hydrocephalus dilates the ventricles proximal to the obstruction.
- The obstructed CSF is under pressure, causing atrophy of the cerebral cortex and degeneration of the white matter tracts. Preservation of gray matter is selective.
- When excess CSF fills a defect caused by atrophy, a degenerative disorder, or a surgical excision, the fluid isn't under pressure and atrophy and degenerative changes aren't induced.

CAUSES

Noncommunicating hydrocephalus

- Aqueduct stenosis
- Arnold-Chiari malformation
- Congenital abnormalities in the ventricular system
- Mass lesion, such as a tumor, that compress one of the structures of the ventricular system

Communicating hydrocephalus

- Adhesions from inflammation, such as with meningitis or subarachnoid hemorrhage
- Cerebral atrophy
- Compression of the subarachnoid space by a mass such as a tumor
- Congenital abnormalities of the subarachnoid space
- Head injury
- High venous pressure within the sagittal sinus

ASSESSMENT FINDINGS

- History that may disclose the cause
- High-pitched, shrill cry; irritability
- Anorexia
- Episodes of projectile vomiting
- Enlarged head clearly disproportionate to the infant's growth

- Head possibly appearing normal in size with bulging fontanels
- Distended scalp veins
- Thin, fragile, and shiny scalp skin
- Underdeveloped neck muscles
- Depression of the roof of the eye orbit
- Displacement of the eyes downward
- Prominent sclera (sunset sign)
- Abnormal leg muscle tone
- Signs of increased ICP

TEST RESULTS

- Skull X-rays show thinning of the skull with separation of sutures and widening of the fontanels in infants.
- Angiography, computed tomography scan, and magnetic resonance imaging show differentiations between hydrocephalus and intracranial lesions and Arnold-Chiari deformity.

TREATMENT

- Shunting of CSF directly from the ventricular system to some point beyond the obstruction
- Small, frequent feedings; slow feedings
- Decreased movement during and immediately after meals
- Possible preoperative and postoperative antibiotics
- Surgical correction (the only treatment for hydrocephalus), including:
  - removal of obstruction to CSF flow
  - implantation of a ventriculoperitoneal shunt to divert CSF flow from the brain's lateral ventricle into the peritoneal cavity
  - with a concurrent abdominal problem, ventriculoatrial shunt to divert CSF flow from the brain's lateral ventricle into the right atrium of the heart

KEY PATIENT OUTCOMES

The patient will:
- maintain adequate ventilation
- develop no signs and symptoms of infection
- maintain and improve current level of consciousness
- develop no signs and symptoms of increased ICP.

NURSING INTERVENTIONS

- Elevate the head of the bed to 30 degrees, or put the infant in an infant seat.
- Assess fontanels for tension or fullness.
- Measure head circumference daily.
- Assess for signs and symptoms of increased ICP.
- Give prescribed oxygen as needed.
- Provide small, frequent feedings.
- Decrease the patient's movement during and immediately after meals.
- Provide meticulous skin care.
- Refer the patient to special education programs as appropriate.

After shunt surgery

- Place the patient on the side opposite the operative site.
- Give prescribed I.V. fluids and analgesics.

 ALERT Monitor the patient for vomiting, which may be an early sign of shunt malfunction.

PATIENT TEACHING

Be sure to cover with the parents:
- the disorder, diagnosis, and treatment
- shunt surgery (including hair loss and the visibility of a mechanical device)
- postoperative shunt care
- signs and symptoms of increased ICP or shunt malfunction
- signs and symptoms of infection
- signs and symptoms of paralytic ileus
- need for periodic shunt surgery to lengthen the shunt as the child grows older.

Hyperbilirubinemia, unconjugated
DESCRIPTION

- Excessive serum bilirubin levels and mild jaundice
- Result of hemolytic processes in the neonate
- Can be physiologic (with jaundice the only symptom) or pathologic (resulting from an underlying disease)

- Common in neonates; more common in males than in females and in White infants than in Black infants
- Potential complications: kernicterus, cerebral palsy, epilepsy, and mental retardation
- Also called *neonatal jaundice*

PATHOPHYSIOLOGY

- As erythrocytes break down at the end of their neonatal life cycle, hemoglobin separates into globin (protein) and heme (iron) fragments.
- Heme fragments form unconjugated (indirect) bilirubin, which binds with albumin for transport to liver cells to conjugate with glucuronide, forming direct bilirubin.
- Because unconjugated bilirubin is fat-soluble and can't be excreted in urine or bile, it may escape to extravascular tissue, especially fatty tissue and the brain, resulting in hyperbilirubinemia.
- Hyperbilirubinemia may develop when:
  - certain factors disrupt conjugation and usurp albumin-binding sites, including drugs (such as aspirin, tranquilizers, and sulfonamides) and conditions (such as hypothermia, anoxia, hypoglycemia, and hypoalbuminemia)
  - decreased hepatic function results in reduced bilirubin conjugation
  - increased erythrocyte production or breakdown results from hemolytic disorders or Rh or ABO incompatibility
  - biliary obstruction or hepatitis results in blockage of normal bile flow
  - maternal enzymes present in breast milk inhibit the infant's glucuronyl-transferase conjugating activity.

CAUSES

See *Onset-related causes of hyperbilirubinemia*, page 110.

ASSESSMENT FINDINGS

- Previous sibling with neonatal jaundice
- Family history of anemia, bile stones, splenectomy, or liver disease
- Maternal illness suggestive of viral or other infection
- Maternal drug intake
- Delayed cord clamping

ONSET-RELATED CAUSES OF HYPERBILIRUBINEMIA

The neonate's age at onset of hyperbilirubinemia may provide clues as to the sources of this jaundice-causing disorder.

Day 1
- Blood type incompatibility (Rh, ABO, other minor blood groups)
- Intrauterine infection (rubella, cytomegalic inclusion body disease, toxoplasmosis, syphilis and, occasionally, such bacteria as *Escherichia coli*, *Staphylococcus*, *Pseudomonas*, *Klebsiella*, *Proteus*, and *Streptococcus*)

Day 2 or 3
- Abnormal red blood cell morphology
- Blood group incompatibilities
- Enclosed hemorrhage (skin bruises, subdural hematoma)
- Heinz body anemia from drugs and toxins (vitamin K3, sodium nitrate)
- Infection (usually from gram-negative bacteria)
- Physiologic jaundice
- Polycythemia
- Red cell enzyme deficiencies (glucose-6-phosphate dehydrogenase, hexokinase)
- Respiratory distress syndrome (hyaline membrane disease)
- Transient neonatal hyperbilirubinemia

Day 4 and 5
- Breast-feeding, respiratory distress syndrome, and maternal diabetes
- Crigler-Najjar syndrome (congenital nonhemolytic icterus)
- Gilbert syndrome

Day 7 and later
- Bile duct atresia
- Choledochal cysts
- Galactosemia
- Infection (usually acquired in neonatal period)
- Herpes simplex
- Hypothyroidism
- Neonatal giant cell hepatitis
- Pyloric stenosis

- Birth trauma with bruising
- Yellowish skin, particularly in the sclerae

TEST RESULTS

■ Serum bilirubin levels are elevated.

TREATMENT

▶ *COLLABORATION If the neonate will receive phototherapy in the home, social services can assist in securing the necessary equipment. Additionally, referrals for home health care nursing and community support would be helpful.*

■ Phototherapy
■ Exchange transfusions
■ Albumin
■ Phenobarbital (rarely used)
■ $Rh_o(D)$ immune globulin (RhoGAM) (to Rh-negative mother)

KEY PATIENT OUTCOMES

The patient will:
■ exhibit normal body temperature
■ maintain normal fluid balance
■ maintain skin integrity
■ have a reduced bilirubin level.

NURSING INTERVENTIONS

■ Reassure the family that most neonates experience some degree of jaundice.
■ Keep emergency equipment available when transfusing blood.
■ Administer $Rh_o(D)$ immune globulin to an Rh-negative mother after amniocentesis or, to prevent hemolytic disease in subsequent infants, to an Rh-negative mother during the third trimester, after the birth of an Rh-positive infant, or after spontaneous or elective abortion.
■ Monitor the neonate for jaundice.
■ Assess serum bilirubin levels as ordered.
■ Monitor vital signs closely.
■ Assess intake and output, especially during treatment.
■ Assess for signs and symptoms of bleeding and associated complications.

PATIENT TEACHING

Be sure to cover with the parents:
- the disorder, diagnosis, and treatment
- that the infant's stool contains some bile and may be greenish
- home phototherapy, if ordered.

Large-for-gestational-age neonate

DESCRIPTION

- Birth weight at or above the 90th percentile on the intrauterine growth chart
- Also called *macrosomia*

PATHOPHYSIOLOGY

- Large-for-gestational-age (LGA) neonates are subjected to an overproduction of growth hormone in utero.
- LGA status places the neonate at risk for:
  - increased incidence of cesarean deliveries, birth trauma, and injury
  - hypoglycemia
  - polycythemia.

CAUSES

- Genetics
  - Male neonates usually larger than females
  - Neonates of large parents usually large
  - Neonates of multiparous women usually larger
- Maternal diabetes
  - High maternal blood glucose levels—stimulus for continued insulin production by the fetus
  - Result of this constant state of hyperglycemia: excessive growth and fat deposition

ASSESSMENT FINDINGS

- Weight generally more than 4,000 g (8 lb 8 oz)
- Plump and full faced

- Fractures or intracranial hemorrhage due to trauma during vaginal delivery
- Immature reflexes
- Possible asymmetry of chest secondary to diaphragmatic paralysis occurring from edema of phrenic nerve

TEST RESULTS

- Blood glucose levels reveal possible hypoglycemia in the neonate.
- Bilirubin levels may be increased.

TREATMENT

- Care similar to that required for a preterm neonate
- Close observation
- Supportive care
- Cardiac and respiratory assessment and assistance with resuscitation, if needed
- Maintenance of fluid and electrolyte balance
- Nutritional support
- Prevention of infection
- Assessment of neurologic status
- Maintenance of body temperature and neutral thermal environment
- Monitoring of renal function
- Emotional support to parents
- Assessment of glucose and bilirubin levels

KEY PATIENT OUTCOMES

The patient will:
- maintain a patent airway and adequate ventilation
- exhibit vital signs within acceptable parameters
- maintain a stable body temperature
- remain free from injury
- demonstrate glucose levels within acceptable levels.

NURSING INTERVENTIONS

- Closely assess all body systems.
- Anticipate the need for endotracheal intubation and mechanical ventilation.

- Administer oxygen as ordered, avoiding concentrations that are too high.
- Monitor transcutaneous oxygen levels or pulse oximetry readings.
- Have emergency resuscitation equipment readily available.
- Administer medications to support cardiac and respiratory function.
- Institute measures to maintain a neutral thermal environment; anticipate the need for an incubator or a radiant warmer.
- Avoid vigorous stroking and rubbing; use firm but gentle touch when handling the neonate.
- Support the head and maintain the extremities close to the body during position changes.
- Monitor fluid and electrolyte balance, assess intake and output, and administer I.V. fluid therapy, as ordered.
- Administer nutritional therapy as ordered; provide nonnutritive sucking via a pacifier as appropriate.
- Provide emotional support and guidance to the family; encourage bonding.
- Allow the family to verbalize their concerns; correct any misconceptions or erroneous information.
- Assist with referrals for supportive services.

PATIENT TEACHING

Be sure to cover with the parents:
- the condition, diagnosis, and treatment
- all procedures and treatments, including rationales
- medications and administration
- necessary follow-up.

Meconium aspiration syndrome
DESCRIPTION

- Aspiration of meconium (the neonate's first feces) into the lungs
- Typically occurs with the first breath or while the neonate is in utero
- Thick, sticky, and greenish black substance; may be seen in the amniotic fluid after 34 weeks' gestation

PATHOPHYSIOLOGY

- Asphyxia in utero leads to increased fetal peristalsis, relaxation of the anal sphincter, passage of meconium into the amniotic fluid, and reflex gasping of amniotic fluid into the lungs.

- Neonates with meconium aspiration syndrome (MAS) increase respiratory efforts to create greater negative intrathoracic pressures and improve air flow to the lungs.
- Hyperinflation, hypoxemia, and acidemia cause increased peripheral vascular resistance.
- Right-to-left shunting commonly follows.
- Meconium creates a ball-valve effect, trapping air in the alveolus and preventing adequate gas exchange.
- Chemical pneumonitis results, causing the alveolar walls and interstitial tissues to thicken, again preventing adequate gas exchange.
- Cardiac efficiency can be compromised from pulmonary hypertension.

CAUSES

- Commonly related to fetal distress during labor
- Risk factors for MAS:
  - Advanced gestational age (greater than 40 weeks)
  - Difficult delivery
  - Fetal distress
  - Intrauterine hypoxia
  - Maternal diabetes
  - Maternal hypertension
  - Poor intrauterine growth

ASSESSMENT FINDINGS

- Fetal hypoxia as indicated by altered fetal activity and heart rate
- Dark greenish staining or streaking of the amniotic fluid noted on rupture of membranes
- Obvious presence of meconium in the amniotic fluid
- Greenish staining of the neonate's skin (if the meconium was passed long before delivery) or placenta
- Signs of distress at delivery, such as the neonate appearing limp, an Apgar score below 6, pallor, cyanosis, and respiratory distress
- Coarse crackles when auscultating the neonate's lungs

TEST RESULTS

- Arterial blood gas analysis shows hypoxemia and decreased pH.

- Chest X-ray may show patches or streaks of meconium in the lungs, air trapping, or hyperinflation.

TREATMENT

- Respiratory assistance via mechanical ventilation
- Maintenance of a neutral thermal environment
- Administration of surfactant and an antibiotic
- Extracorporeal membrane oxygenation (in severe cases)

KEY PATIENT OUTCOMES

The patient will:
- maintain a patent airway
- exhibit adequate ventilation and perfusion
- maintain thermoregulation
- remain free from infection.

NURSING INTERVENTIONS

- During labor, continuously monitor the fetus for signs and symptoms of distress.
- Immediately inspect any fluid passed with rupture of the membranes.
- Assist with immediate endotracheal suctioning before the first breaths, as indicated.
- Monitor lung status closely, including breath sounds and respiratory rate and character.
- Frequently assess the neonate's vital signs.
- Administer treatment modalities, such as oxygen and respiratory support, as ordered.
- Institute measures to maintain a neutral thermal environment.
- Provide the family with emotional support and guidance.

PATIENT TEACHING

Be sure to cover with the parents:
- the disorder, diagnosis, and treatment
- procedures being used
- medications
- potential complications.

Necrotizing enterocolitis

DESCRIPTION

- Inflammatory disease of the GI mucosa involving mucosal or transmucosal necrosis of part of the intestine
- Most commonly occurs in preterm neonates, usually 3 to 10 days after birth
- Occurs in any portion of the bowel; most commonly the distal ileum and the proximal colon

PATHOPHYSIOLOGY

- Necrotizing enterocolitis (NEC) is associated with three events: perinatal hypoxia, bacterial invasion, and high-solute feedings.
- Blood flow to the gastric mucosa is decreased as a result of the shunting of blood to vital organs secondary to perinatal hypoxia.
- Mucosal cells lining the bowel wall die.
- Protective, lubricating mucus isn't secreted.
- The bowel wall is attacked by proteolytic enzymes.
- The bowel wall swells and breaks down.
- Bacteria invade, and concentrated feedings provide a source for the bacteria to grow.

CAUSES

- Exact cause unknown; appears to occur in neonates whose GI tract suffered vascular compromise or infection
- Prenatal factors: preterm labor, prolonged rupture of membranes, preeclampsia, maternal sepsis, amnionitis, and uterine hypoxia
- Postnatal factors: respiratory distress syndrome, patent ductus arteriosus, congenital heart disease, exchange transfusion, low birth weight, low Apgar scores, umbilical catheterization, hypothermia, GI infection, hypoglycemia, and asphyxia

ASSESSMENT FINDINGS

- Distended abdomen
- Gastric retention
- Blood in the stool or gastric contents

- Lethargy
- Poor feeding
- Vomiting
- Hypotension
- Apnea

TEST RESULTS

- Radiography may show intestinal dilation and free air in the abdomen (indicating perforation).
- Blood studies may show anemia, leukopenia, leukocytosis, and electrolyte imbalances.

TREATMENT

▶ **COLLABORATION** *The neonate with NEC may require multidisciplinary care. Surgical specialists may be involved if intestinal necrosis or perforation (free air in the abdomen on X-ray) occurs. If surgery results in the possible creation of an ostomy, enterostomal therapy would be indicated. Nutritional specialists assist in determining the neonate's nutritional needs and in planning appropriate therapy. Social services would be involved to help with emotional support and guidance, financial concerns, and home care and community referrals as part of discharge planning.*

- Prevention
- Discontinuation of enteral feedings
- Nasogastric (NG) suction
- Administration of I.V. antibiotics
- Administration of parenteral fluids
- Surgery

KEY PATIENT OUTCOMES

The patient will:
- maintain a patent airway
- maintain normal fluid and electrolyte balance
- remain free from infection
- exhibit vital signs within acceptable parameters
- maintain adequate weight.

NURSING INTERVENTIONS

- Maintain nothing-by-mouth status, and institute gastric suctioning, as ordered.
- Administer I.V. fluid therapy as ordered.

ALERT *Assess the abdomen frequently, including palpating for tenderness and rigidity, auscultating bowel sounds, and measuring abdominal girth. Inspect the abdominal area for redness or shininess, which could indicate peritonitis.*

- Test stools, vomitus, and gastric drainage for blood.
- Carefully monitor intake and output and serum electrolyte levels.
- Administer analgesics, as ordered, for evidence of pain.
- Maintain infection control measures, with an emphasis on careful hand washing.
- Provide support to the patient and family throughout medical or surgical interventions.
- Encourage family interaction with the neonate.
- Provide referrals to appropriate community resources for support and guidance.

PATIENT TEACHING

Be sure to cover with the parents:
- the disorder, diagnosis, and treatment
- therapies used such as NG suctioning
- preoperative and postoperative interventions, if indicated
- potential complications
- feeding measures when appropriate
- community sources of support
- necessary follow-up.

 Life-threatening disorder

Neonatal sepsis
DESCRIPTION

- Occurrence of pathogenic microorganisms or their toxins in the blood or tissues
- Can occur before, during, or after delivery

PATHOPHYSIOLOGY

- The neonate is susceptible to infections because his immune system is immature and slow to react.
- The antibodies the neonate received from his mother during pregnancy and currently receives from breast milk help protect him from invading organisms; time is needed to reach optimum levels, which affects the protection provided.
- Pathogenic organisms cross the placenta into the fetal circulatory system or ascend up from the vagina and begin to multiply.
- The neonate is exposed to organisms from an infected birth canal during the birthing process.
- The pathologic organism overcomes the neonate's defenses, leading to infection and sepsis.

CAUSES

- Any bacteria, virus, or fungus
- Most commonly, gram-negative *Escherichia coli, Aerobacter,* and *Klebsiella* and gram-positive beta-hemolytic streptococci
- Prolonged rupture of membranes

ASSESSMENT FINDINGS

- Subtle, nonspecific behavioral changes, such as lethargy and hypotonia
- Temperature instability
- Feeding pattern changes, such as poor sucking and decreased intake
- Apnea
- Hyperbilirubinemia
- Abdominal distention
- Skin color changes, including mottling, pallor, and cyanosis

TEST RESULTS

- Blood cultures are positive for the causative organism.
- Complete blood count reveals the presence or absence of anemia, leukopenia, severe or absent neutropenia and, usually, thrombocytopenia.
- Arterial blood gas analysis shows increased blood pH and partial pres-

sure of arterial oxygen and decreased partial pressure of arterial carbon dioxide.

■ Oxygen saturation is less than 94%.

TREATMENT

▶ **COLLABORATION** *Caring for the neonate with sepsis requires a multidisciplinary approach. An infectious disease specialist may be involved to identify the causative organism and determine and coordinate antimicrobial therapy. A dietitian may assist in managing the neonate's metabolic needs and administration of nutrition. Respiratory and renal specialists may be involved if the neonate develops respiratory or renal complications. A social services referral may be needed to provide support for the parents and assist with community referrals.*

■ Lumbar puncture to rule out meningitis
■ Urine, skin, blood, and nasopharyngeal cultures
■ Gastric aspiration
■ Antibiotic administration

KEY PATIENT OUTCOMES

The patient will:

■ maintain adequate ventilation
■ maintain adequate cardiac output
■ demonstrate vital signs within acceptable parameters
■ maintain adequate fluid volume and weight
■ demonstrate resolving signs and symptoms of infection.

NURSING INTERVENTIONS

■ Collect specimens to identify the causative organism.
■ Assess the neonate's vital signs once per hour or more frequently, as indicated.
■ Expect to administer a broad-spectrum antibiotic before culture results are received and to switch to specific antibiotic therapy after results are received.
■ Provide supportive care, including maintenance of a neutral thermal environment.

- Administer nutritional support.
- Assist with respiratory support measures, including oxygen therapy as ordered.
- Monitor fluid and electrolyte balance; administer I.V. fluid therapy as ordered.
- Institute measures to provide cardiovascular support as needed.
- Provide support to the family; encourage them to verbalize their feelings and to interact with the neonate.

PATIENT TEACHING

Be sure to cover with the parents:
- the disorder, diagnosis, and treatment
- equipment and procedures, including their purpose
- medications used
- possible complications
- necessary follow-up.

Phenylketonuria

DESCRIPTION

- A rare hereditary condition, considered an inborn metabolic error
- A disease of protein metabolism characterized by the inability of the body to metabolize the essential amino acid phenylalanine

PATHOPHYSIOLOGY

- Persons with phenylketonuria (PKU) have almost no activity of phenylalanine hydroxylase, an enzyme that helps convert phenylalanine to tyrosine.
- As a result, phenylalanine accumulates in the blood and urine and tyrosine levels are low.
- Phenylalanine and its abnormal metabolites accumulate in the brain.
- This accumulation affects the normal development of the brain and central nervous system (CNS).
- Tyrosine is needed to form the pigment melanin and the hormones epinephrine and thyroxine.

- Decreased melanin production results in the similar fair appearance of children with PKU.
- CNS damage can be minimized if treatment is initiated before age 3 months; mental retardation can occur if the condition is untreated.

CAUSES

- Genetic; inherited as an autosomal recessive trait in which both parents must pass the gene on for the child to be affected

ASSESSMENT FINDINGS

- Failure to thrive
- Vomiting
- Rashes and eczematous skin lesions
- Decreased pigmentation
- Seizures and tremors
- Microcephaly
- Hyperactivity and irritability
- Purposeless, repetitive motions
- Musty odor from skin and urinary excretion of phenylacetic acid

TEST RESULTS

- Guthrie test result is positive.
- Guthrie heelstick blood test is required by most states. The test should be performed at least 24 hours after initiation of feedings.

TREATMENT

- Low-phenylalanine formula (such as Lofenalac)
- Continued special diet that limits phenylalanine intake

KEY PATIENT OUTCOMES

The patient will:
- demonstrate adequate weight gain
- ingest adequate nutrition within restrictions
- demonstrate growth and development appropriate for age.

PHENYLALANINE IN FOODS

The neonate's diet should meet his nutritional needs for optimum growth while maintaining a safe phenylalanine level (2 to 8 mg/dl). Phenylalanine levels greater than 10 to 15 mg/dl can lead to brain damage; levels lower than 2 mg/dl can lead to protein catabolism and growth retardation.

Specialized formulas, such as Lofenalac, are available. In addition, foods with low levels of phenylalanine include:

- vegetables
- fruits
- juices
- some cereals, breads, and starches.

Foods that should be avoided because of their high phenylalanine content include:

- dairy products
- eggs
- meat
- foods and drinks containing aspartame (NutraSweet).

NURSING INTERVENTIONS

- Provide low-phenylalanine formula for the neonate.
- Inform the family about the neonate's need for limited phenylalanine intake.
- Provide the family with a list of foods to allow in the neonate's diet as well as those to avoid.
- Offer emotional support to the family (Because the disorder is genetic, the parents may feel responsible.)

PATIENT TEACHING

Be sure to cover with the parents:

- the disorder, diagnosis, and treatment
- genetic transmission
- dietary measures, including foods high and low in phenylalanine (see *Phenylalanine in foods*)
- meal planning
- monitoring of blood levels
- necessary follow-up.

Preterm neonate

DESCRIPTION

■ Delivery of a neonate before the end of the 37th week of gestation
■ Associated with numerous problems because all body systems are immature
■ Preterm neonates between 24 and 37 weeks' gestation demonstrating the best chance of survival

PATHOPHYSIOLOGY

■ Preterm delivery may occur because of maternal disease that necessitates delivery of the neonate for the health of the mother — for example, preeclampsia.
■ Preterm delivery may also be a direct result of preterm labor.

CAUSES

■ Associated with maternal risk factors:
  – Adolescent pregnancy
  – Cervical insufficiency
  – Gestational hypertension
  – High, unexplained alpha fetoprotein level in second trimester
  – Lack of prenatal care
  – Multiple pregnancy
  – Placenta previa
  – Premature rupture of membranes
  – Previous preterm delivery
  – Substance abuse
  – Uterine abnormalities
■ Underlying condition that results in the delivery of the neonate before term

ASSESSMENT FINDINGS

■ Low birth weight
■ Minimal subcutaneous fat deposits
■ Proportionally large head in relation to body
■ Prominent sucking pads in the cheeks
■ Wrinkled features

- Thin, smooth, shiny skin that's almost translucent
- Veins clearly visible under the thin, transparent epidermis
- Lanugo hair over the body
- Sparse, fine, fuzzy hair on the head
- Soft, pliable ear cartilage (the ear may fold easily)
- Minimal creases in the soles and palms
- Prominent eyes, possibly closed
- Few scrotal rugae (males)
- Undescended testes (males)
- Prominent labia and clitoris (females)
- Inactivity (although may be unusually active immediately after birth)
- Extension of extremities
- Absence of suck reflex
- Weak swallow, gag, and cough reflexes
- Weak grasp reflex
- Ability to bring the neonate's elbow across the chest when eliciting the scarf sign
- Ability to easily bring the neonate's heel to his ear
- Inability to maintain body temperature
- Limited ability to excrete solutes in urine
- Increased susceptibility to infection, hyperbilirubinemia, and hypoglycemia
- Periodic breathing, hypoventilation, and periods of apnea

TEST RESULTS

- Chest X-rays may reveal underlying pulmonary problems.
- Echocardiography may reveal cardiac dysfunction.
- Arterial blood gas analysis reveals possible hypoxemia and acid-base abnormalities.
- Serum electrolytes reveal possible imbalances.
- Serum glucose levels may be decreased, indicating hypoglycemia.

TREATMENT

COLLABORATION *The preterm neonate requires a multidisciplinary approach to care because all body systems are immature and the neonate is at risk for numerous complications in any body system. Pulmonary and cardiac specialists may be involved in maintaining adequate cardiac output and ventilation. If renal*

*or GI dysfunction occurs, specialists in these areas may be enlist-
ed. Nutritional support is also essential. Because of the critical
nature of the neonate's status, social services may be involved to
provide emotional support to the family and to assist with long-
term planning and follow-up.*

- Cardiac and respiratory assessment and assistance
- Resuscitation, if needed
- Maintenance of fluid and electrolyte balance
- Nutritional support
- Prevention of infection
- Assessment of neurologic status
- Maintenance of body temperature and a neutral thermal environment
- Monitoring of renal function
- Emotional support to the family
- Assessment of glucose and bilirubin levels

KEY PATIENT OUTCOMES

The patient will:
- maintain thermoregulation
- maintain adequate ventilation, perfusion, and cardiac output
- remain free from injury
- demonstrate intake of adequate nutrients to support metabolic
  demands and growth
- demonstrate an increase in weight
- exhibit appropriate behavioral responses
- remain free from infection.

NURSING INTERVENTIONS

- Closely assess all body systems.
- Anticipate the need for endotracheal intubation and mechanical venti-
  lation.
- Administer oxygen as ordered, avoiding concentrations that are too
  high.
- Monitor transcutaneous oxygen levels or pulse oximetry readings.
- Have emergency resuscitation equipment readily available.
- Administer medications to support cardiac and respiratory function.
- Institute measures to maintain a neutral thermal environment; antici-
  pate the need for an incubator or a radiant warmer.

- Avoid vigorous stroking and rubbing; use a firm but gentle touch when handling the neonate.
- Support the head and maintain extremities close to the body during position changes.
- Monitor fluid and electrolyte balance, assess intake and output, and administer I.V. fluid therapy, as ordered.
- Administer nutritional therapy as ordered.

   ALERT *Neonates born before 34 weeks' gestation have uncoordinated sucking and swallowing reflexes; therefore, gavage or I.V. feeding may be necessary. Provide nonnutritive sucking using a pacifier as appropriate.*

- Provide emotional support and guidance to the family, allow them to verbalize their concerns, and correct any misconceptions or erroneous information.
- Assist with referrals for supportive services.

PATIENT TEACHING

Be sure to cover with the parents:
- the disorder, diagnosis, and treatment
- procedures, equipment, and medications being used
- possible complications and risks
- nutritional needs
- methods to promote bonding and attachment
- expectations for growth and development
- necessary follow-up.

 Life-threatening disorder

Respiratory distress syndrome
DESCRIPTION

- Respiratory disorder that involves widespread alveolar collapse
- Most common cause of neonatal death
- If mild, subsides slowly after about 3 days
- Incidence: typically, neonates born before the 27th gestational week; about 60% of those born before the 28th week
- Risk factors: cesarean delivery, mother with diabetes, delivery after antepartum hemorrhage

COMPLICATIONS THAT MAY AFFECT PRETERM NEONATES

Because of the preterm neonate's fragile condition and the numerous treatments and procedures typically needed, stay alert for these complications:

- respiratory distress syndrome
- intraventricular hemorrhage
- retinopathy of prematurity
- patent ductus arteriosus
- necrotizing enterocolitis
- bronchopulmonary dysplasia
- apnea of prematurity.

- Also called *RDS* or *hyaline membrane disease* (see *Complications that may affect preterm neonates*)

PATHOPHYSIOLOGY

- RDS is characterized by poor gas exchange and ventilatory failure due to a lack of surfactant in the lungs.
- Surfactant is a phospholipid secreted by the alveolar epithelium.
- It coats the alveoli, keeping them open so gas exchange can occur.
- In preterm neonates, the lungs may not be fully developed and therefore may not have sufficient surfactant available.
- Inability to maintain alveolar stability results.
- The lack of surfactant leads to atelectasis, labored breathing, respiratory acidosis, and hypoxemia.
- With worsening atelectasis, pulmonary vascular resistance increases, which decreases blood flow to the lungs.
- Right-to-left shunting of blood perpetuates fetal circulation by keeping the foramen ovale and ductus arteriosus patent.
- The alveoli can become necrotic, and the capillaries are damaged.
- Ischemia allows fluid to leak into the interstitial and alveolar spaces, and a hyaline membrane forms.
- This membrane greatly hinders respiratory function by decreasing the compliance of the lungs.
- Hypoxia and acidosis result.
- Compensatory grunting occurs, producing positive end-expiratory pressure (PEEP) that helps prevent further alveolar collapse.

CAUSES

- Surfactant deficiency stemming from preterm birth

ASSESSMENT FINDINGS

- History of preterm birth or cesarean birth
- Maternal history of diabetes or antepartum hemorrhage
- Rapid, shallow respirations
- Intercostal, subcostal, or sternal retractions
- Nasal flaring
- Audible expiratory grunting
- Pallor
- Frothy sputum
- Low body temperature
- Diminished air entry and crackles
- Possible hypotension, peripheral edema, and oliguria
- Possible apnea, bradycardia, and cyanosis

TEST RESULTS

- Arterial blood gas (ABG) analysis shows decreased partial pressure of arterial oxygen (Pao_2) and arterial pH; partial pressure of arterial carbon dioxide may be normal, decreased, or increased.
- Lecithin-sphingomyelin ratio shows prenatal lung development and RDS risk.
- Chest X-rays may show a fine reticulonodular pattern and dark streaks, indicating air-filled, dilated bronchioles.

TREATMENT

▶ *COLLABORATION The neonate with RDS is critically ill and needs the services of a neonatal intensive care unit. Pulmonary specialists and respiratory therapy most likely will be involved to assist in maintaining the neonate's ventilation and perfusion. Nutritional specialists can assist in promoting adequate nutrition to support the neonate's increased metabolic demands and to promote optimal growth and development. Social services and pastoral care specialists may be needed for family support.*

- Aggressive management, assisted by mechanical ventilation with PEEP or continuous positive airway pressure (CPAP) administered by a tight-fitting face mask or, when necessary, an endotracheal tube
- For a neonate who can't maintain adequate gas exchange, high-frequency oscillation ventilation
- Radiant warmer or Isolette
- Warm, humidified, oxygen-enriched gases given by oxygen hood or mechanical ventilation
- Tube feedings or total parenteral nutrition
- I.V. fluids and sodium bicarbonate
- Pancuronium bromide (Pavulon)
- Prophylactic antibiotics
- Diuretics
- Surfactant replacement therapy
- Vitamin E
- Antenatal corticosteroids
- Possible tracheostomy

KEY PATIENT OUTCOMES

The patient will:
- maintain adequate ventilation
- maintain a patent airway
- remain free from infection
- maintain skin integrity.

NURSING INTERVENTIONS

- Monitor vital signs closely for changes; use an Isolette or a radiant warmer.
- Assess skin color and integrity; report signs of decreased peripheral circulation.
- Assess cardiopulmonary status for changes; auscultate lung sounds for abnormalities.
- Administer oxygen as ordered.
- Monitor results of pulse oximetry every 1 to 2 hours, and evaluate ABG results, as ordered.

  ALERT *Watch for evidence of complications from oxygen therapy: lung capillary damage, decreased mucus flow, impaired ciliary functioning, and widespread atelectasis. Also stay* *alert for signs of patent ductus arteriosus, heart failure, retinopathy, pulmonary hypertension, necrotizing enterocolitis, and neurologic abnormalities.*

- Measure daily weight, and monitor intake and output.
- Give prescribed drugs as ordered.
- Check the umbilical catheter for arterial or venous hypotension as appropriate.
- Suction as needed.
- Change the transcutaneous Pao_2 monitor lead placement site every 2 to 4 hours.
- Adjust PEEP or CPAP settings as indicated by ABG values.

ALERT *In a neonate on a mechanical ventilator, watch carefully for signs of barotrauma and accidental disconnection from the ventilator. Check ventilator settings frequently. Stay alert for signs of complications of PEEP or CPAP therapy, such as decreased cardiac output, pneumothorax, and pneumomediastinum.*

- Provide parenteral nutrition and avoid gavage and oral feedings during the acute stage of the disease because these interventions increase respiratory rate and oxygen consumption.
- Cluster nursing activities to provide the neonate with rest periods; disturb the neonate with RDS as little as possible.
- Implement measures to prevent infection.
- Provide skin and mouth care every 2 hours.
- Encourage the family to participate in the neonate's care.
- Offer emotional support; encourage the family to ask questions and to express their fears and concerns.
- Advise them that full recovery may take up to 12 months.
- Refer the family to pastoral counselors and a social worker as indicated.
- Refer the neonate for follow-up care with a neonatal ophthalmologist as indicated.

PATIENT TEACHING

Be sure to cover with the parents:
- the disorder, diagnosis, and treatment
- procedures, treatments, and drugs, including possible adverse effects

- explanations of respiratory equipment, alarm sounds, and mechanical noise
- potential complications
- when to notify the health care provider.

Retinopathy of prematurity

DESCRIPTION

- Alteration in vision leading to partial or total blindness
- Can cause mild to severe eye and vision problems

PATHOPHYSIOLOGY

- High oxygen concentrations lead to vasoconstriction of immature retinal blood vessels.
- Fluctuating oxygen administration levels lead to rapid vasodilation and vasoconstriction of immature, fragile retinal blood vessels.
- Subsequent rupture of vessels occurs with partial or complete retinal detachment.

CAUSES

- Preterm birth
- Supplemental oxygen; typically prolonged exposure to high concentrations of oxygen or fluctuations in oxygen administration levels

ASSESSMENT FINDINGS

- Retinal changes revealed by ophthalmologic examination

TEST RESULTS

- No significant results; diagnosis is based on ophthalmologic examination.

TREATMENT

- Monitoring of oxygen concentration
- Monitoring of arterial blood gas (ABG) levels

- Monitoring of transcutaneous oxygen levels and pulse oximetry
- Ophthalmologic examinations at regular intervals during and after hospitalization
- Administration of vitamin E (reduces incidence of retinopathy of prematurity by modifying tissues' response to effects of oxygen)
- Cryosurgery or laser surgery

KEY PATIENT OUTCOMES

The patient will:
- maintain optimal vision
- remain free from injury.

NURSING INTERVENTIONS

- Closely monitor oxygen concentration levels being administered; obtain transcutaneous oxygen and ABG levels and pulse oximetry readings, as ordered.
- Administer oxygen carefully, ensuring that the lowest concentration necessary is being used.
- Provide preoperative and postoperative care as indicated.
- Offer emotional support and guidance, including referrals for community support, if needed.

PATIENT TEACHING

Be sure to cover with the parents:
- the disorder, diagnosis, and treatment
- surgery, if indicated
- need for follow-up eye examinations
- available community support services.

Small-for-gestational-age neonate
DESCRIPTION

- Birth weight at or below the 10th percentile on the intrauterine growth chart
- Neonate may be premature, term, or postmature

- Risks:
  - Perinatal asphyxia
  - Hypoglycemia
  - Hypocalcemia
  - Aspiration syndromes
  - Increased heat loss
  - Feeding difficulties
  - Polycythemia
- Also called *small for date* and *intrauterine growth restriction*

PATHOPHYSIOLOGY

- Fetus doesn't receive the required nutrition to support growth.
- Subsequently, the rate of growth doesn't meet the expected growth pattern.

CAUSES

- Conditions in the fetus that may also contribute to the birth of a small-for-gestational-age (SGA) neonate:
  - Chromosomal abnormalities and malformations
  - Intrauterine infection
- Conditions in the mother that may contribute to the birth of an SGA neonate:
  - Advanced diabetes
  - Age older than 35
  - Drug use
  - Gestational hypertension
  - Poor nutrition
  - Smoking
- Partial placental separation and malfunction also possible contributors
- Underlying problem: intrauterine growth restriction

ASSESSMENT FINDINGS

- Wide-eyed look
- Sunken abdomen
- Loose, dry skin
- Decreased chest and abdomen circumferences
- Decreased subcutaneous fat

- Thin, dry umbilical cord
- Sparse scalp hair

TEST RESULTS

- Blood glucose levels may reveal hypoglycemia.
- Red blood cell count may be increased.

TREATMENT

- Supportive care
- Nutritional support

KEY PATIENT OUTCOMES

The patient will:
- maintain a patent airway and adequate ventilation
- exhibit vital signs within acceptable parameters
- maintain a stable body temperature
- remain free from injury
- demonstrate glucose levels within acceptable levels.

NURSING INTERVENTIONS

- Support respiratory efforts, monitor respiratory status closely for changes, and institute respiratory care measures, as indicated by the neonate's condition.
- Institute measures to provide a neutral thermal environment.
- Protect the neonate from infection.
- Provide appropriate nutrition; keep in mind that SGA neonates have higher caloric needs and benefit from frequent feedings.

   ALERT Monitor blood glucose levels as ordered. Hypo-glycemia is common because of reduced glycogen stores. I.V. glucose may be needed if blood glucose levels are lower than 40 mg/dl.

- Maintain adequate hydration, monitor intake and output, and administer I.V. fluid therapy as ordered.
- Cluster nursing care activities.
- Provide meticulous skin care.

- Facilitate growth and development; encourage family interaction with the neonate to promote bonding.
- Keep the family informed and provide emotional support.
- Assist with referrals for supportive services.

PATIENT TEACHING

Be sure to cover with the parents:
- the condition, diagnosis, and treatment
- all procedures and treatments, including rationales
- necessary follow-up.

 Life-threatening disorder

Tracheoesophageal fistula
DESCRIPTION

- A developmental anomaly characterized by an abnormal connection between the trachea and esophagus
- Usually accompanies esophageal atresia, in which the esophagus is closed off at some point
- Most common malformation: esophageal atresia with fistula to the distal segment
- Requires immediate diagnosis and correction
- Potential complications: aspiration of secretions into the lungs, leading to respiratory distress, pneumonia, or cessation of breathing
- Postoperative complications: abnormal esophageal motility, recurrent fistulas, pneumothorax, and esophageal stricture

PATHOPHYSIOLOGY

- Tracheoesophageal fistula and esophageal atresia result from the failure of the embryonic esophagus and trachea to develop and separate correctly.
- Respiratory system development begins at about day 26 of gestation.
- Abnormal development of the septum during this time can lead to tracheoesophageal fistula.
- The most common abnormality is type C tracheoesophageal fistula with esophageal atresia, in which the upper section of the esophagus

terminates in a blind pouch and the lower section ascends from the
stomach and connects with the trachea by a short fistulous tract. (See
Types of tracheoesophageal anomalies.)

- In type A atresia, both esophageal segments are blind pouches and neither is connected to the airway.
- In types B and D, the upper portion of the esophagus opens into the
  trachea; infants with this anomaly may experience life-threatening aspiration of saliva or food.
- In type E (or H-type) tracheoesophageal fistula without atresia, the fistula may occur anywhere between the level of the cricoid cartilage and
  the midesophagus but usually is higher in the trachea than in the
  esophagus. Such a fistula may be as small as a pinpoint.

CAUSES

- Commonly found in infants with other anomalies, including:
  - congenital heart disease
  - genitourinary abnormalities
  - imperforate anus
  - intestinal atresia
- Congenital anomalies

ASSESSMENT FINDINGS

- Coughing and choking after eating
- Respiratory distress
- Drooling
- Immediate aspiration of saliva into the airway and bacterial pneumoni-
  tis (type B [proximal fistula] and type D [fistula to both segments])
- Repeated episodes of pneumonitis, pulmonary infection, and abdomi-
  nal infection; choking followed by cyanosis (type E [or H-type])
- Normal swallowing, excessive drooling, and possible respiratory dis-
  tress (type A)
- Seemingly normal swallowing followed shortly afterward by coughing,
  struggling, cyanosis, and lack of breathing (type C)

TEST RESULTS

- Chest X-rays demonstrate the position of the catheter and can also
  show a dilated, air-filled upper esophageal pouch, pneumonia in the

FOCUS IN
TYPES OF TRACHEOESOPHAGEAL ANOMALIES

Congenital malformations of the esophagus occur in about 1 in 4,000 live births. The American Academy of Pediatrics classifies the anatomic variations of tracheo-esophageal anomaly as follows:

- type A (7.7%) — esophageal atresia without fistula
- type B (0.8%) — esophageal atresia with tracheoesopha-geal fistula to the proximal segment
- type C (86.5%) — esophageal atresia with fistula to the distal segment
- type D (0.7%) — esophageal atresia with fistula to both segments
- type E (or H-type) (4.2%) — tracheoesophageal fistula without atresia.

TYPE A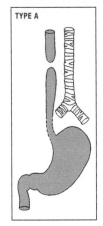

TYPE B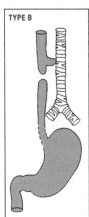

TYPE C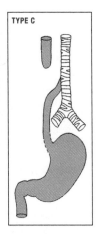

TYPE D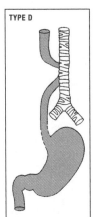

TYPE E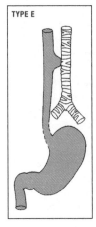

right upper lobe, or bilateral pneumonitis. Pneumonia and pneumonitis suggest aspiration.

- Abdominal X-rays show gas in the bowel in a distal fistula (type C) but none in a proximal fistula (type B) or in atresia without fistula (type A).
- Cinefluorography allows visualization on a fluoroscopic screen. After a size 10 or 12 French catheter is passed through the patient's nostril into the esophagus, a small amount of contrast medium is instilled to define the tip of the upper pouch and to differentiate between overflow aspiration from a blind end (atresia) and aspiration from passage of liquids through a tracheoesophageal fistula.
- A size 6 or 8 French catheter passed through the nose meets an obstruction (esophageal atresia) about 4″ to 5″ (10 to 12.5 cm) distal to the nostrils. Aspirate of gastric contents is less acidic than normal.

TREATMENT

COLLABORATION The neonate with tracheoesophageal fistula requires multidisciplinary care. Surgery is necessary to repair the anomaly. Pulmonary specialists and respiratory therapists may be required to manage the neonate's oxygenation, including treatment related to possible aspiration. A GI specialist may collaborate with the pulmonary specialist for ventilatory management. Nutritional therapy is indicated to ensure adequate intake and promote growth. Social services are important for assisting with financial concerns, providing emotional support, planning for discharge (including evaluating the need for home health nursing), and assisting with follow-up examinations and testing.

- Administer I.V. fluids as ordered.
- Place the patient in a supine position with the head low to facilitate drainage or with the head elevated to prevent aspiration.
- After surgery, assist with placement of a suction catheter in the upper esophageal pouch to control secretions and prevent aspiration.
- Administer antibiotics for superimposed infection.
- Tracheoesophageal fistula and esophageal atresia require surgical correction and are usually surgical emergencies. The type and timing of the surgical procedure depend on the nature of the anomaly, the patient's general condition, and the presence of coexisting congenital defects.

- In premature neonates (nearly 33% of neonates with this anomaly) who are poor surgical risks, correction of combined tracheoesophageal fistula and esophageal atresia is done in two stages: first, gastrostomy (for gastric decompression, prevention of reflux, and feeding) and closure of the fistula; then, 1 to 2 months later, anastomosis of the esophagus.
- Correction of esophageal atresia alone requires anastomosis of the proximal and distal esophageal segments in one or two stages. End-to-end anastomosis commonly produces postoperative stricture; end-to-side anastomosis is less likely to do so.
- If the esophageal ends are widely separated, treatment may include a colonic interposition (grafting a piece of the colon) or elongation of the proximal segment of the esophagus by bougienage.

KEY PATIENT OUTCOMES

The patient will:
- remain free from respiratory complications
- demonstrate hemodynamic stability.

NURSING INTERVENTIONS

- Assess respiratory status closely; administer oxygen as needed.
- Perform pulmonary physiotherapy and suctioning as needed.
- Provide a humid environment.
- Administer antibiotics and parenteral fluids.
- Maintain gastrostomy tube feedings.
- Monitor intake and output.
- Provide preoperative and postoperative care.
- Assess the function of chest tubes postoperatively.
- After surgery, monitor the neonate for signs and symptoms of complications.
- Offer the family support and guidance in dealing with their infant's acute illness.
- Encourage them to participate in care and to hold and touch the infant as much as possible.
- Inform the family that X-rays are required about 10 days after surgery, and again 1 and 3 months later, to evaluate the effectiveness of surgical repair.

PATIENT TEACHING

Be sure to cover with the parents:
- the disorder, diagnosis, and treatment
- feeding procedures
- recognizing and reporting complications
- proper positioning.
- necessary follow-up care, including diagnostic tests.

Transient tachypnea of the neonate
DESCRIPTION

- A mild respiratory problem in neonates, typically beginning after birth and generally lasting about 2 days
- Also called *type II respiratory distress syndrome, wet lung,* or *TTN*

PATHOPHYSIOLOGY

- Before birth, the fetal lungs are filled with amniotic fluid.
- All of the fetus's nutrients and oxygen come from the mother through the placenta; the fetus doesn't use his lungs to breathe.
- During the birth process, some of the neonate's lung fluid is squeezed out as he passes through the birth canal.
- After birth, the remaining fluid is pushed out of the lungs as the lungs fill with air.
- Any fluid that remains is later expelled by coughing or reabsorbed into the bloodstream.
- TTN results from aspiration of amniotic or tracheal fluid are compounded either by delayed clearing of the airway or by excess fluid entering the lungs.
- TNN spontaneously fades as lung fluid is absorbed, usually by 48 hours of life, as respiratory activity becomes effective.
- After TTN resolves, the neonate usually recovers completely and has no increased risk of further respiratory problems.

CAUSES

- Commonly observed in neonates born by cesarean birth because these

neonates don't receive the thoracic compression that helps to expel fluid during vaginal delivery
- Results from delayed absorption of fetal lung fluid after birth
- Additional risk factors:
  - Neonates of mothers who smoked during pregnancy
  - Neonates of diabetic mothers
  - Neonates who are small for gestational age
  - Neonates who are small or premature, or who were born rapidly by vaginal delivery (may not have received effective squeezing of the thorax to remove fetal lung fluid)

ASSESSMENT FINDINGS

- Increased respiratory rate (greater than 60 breaths/minute)
- Expiratory grunting
- Nasal flaring
- Slight cyanosis
- Retractions
- Tachypnea

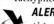 **ALERT** *Increased carbon dioxide levels may be a sign of fatigue and impending respiratory failure.*

TEST RESULTS

- Chest X-ray, the diagnostic standard for TTN, reveals streaking (correlates with lymphatic engorgement of retained fetal lung fluid).
- Arterial blood gas analysis may indicate hypoxemia and decreased carbon dioxide levels.
- Complete blood count may show infection.
- Pulse oximetry reveals oxygen saturation of less than 94%.

TREATMENT

- Oxygen administration
- Ventilatory assistance (rarely needed)
- Maintenance of acid-base balance
- Thermoregulation
- Adequate nutrition via gavage feedings or I.V. fluids
- Transcutaneous oxygen monitoring
- Protection from infection

KEY PATIENT OUTCOMES

The patient will:
- maintain a patent airway and ventilation
- remain free from infection
- maintain adequate nutrition
- maintain a stable body temperature.

NURSING INTERVENTIONS

- Closely monitor the neonate's heart rate, respiratory rate, and oxygenation status.
- Provide respiratory support, including mechanical ventilation, if necessary.
- Institute measures to maintain a neutral thermal environment.
- Minimize stimulation by decreasing lights and noise levels.
- Provide nutritional support via gavage feedings or parenteral nutrition.

    ALERT *The neonate with TTN has difficulty with oral feedings because of increased respiratory rate and increased work of breathing related to coordination of neonatal mechanisms of sucking, swallowing, and breathing. Monitor closely, especially during feedings, because neonates with TTN are at high risk for aspiration because of their rapid respiratory rate.*

- Provide emotional support to the family.

PATIENT TEACHING

Be sure to cover with the parents:
- the disorder, diagnosis, and treatment
- gavage feedings
- time frame for resolution with no increased risk of respiratory problems
- necessary follow-up.

Part two

Treatments

Amnioinfusion

DESCRIPTION

- Replacement of amniotic fluid volume through intrauterine infusion
- Involves the use of an isotonic solution, such as normal saline or lactated Ringer's solution, via a pressure catheter

PURPOSE

- Indicated when umbilical cord compression is a factor or when repetitive variable decelerations aren't alleviated by maternal position change and oxygen administration
- May also be done to dilute meconium before aspiration occurs
- Helps to relieve umbilical cord compression in such conditions as oligohydramnios associated with postmaturity, intrauterine growth retardation, and premature rupture of membranes

PATIENT PREPARATION

- Explain the procedure and the rationale for its use.
- Prepare the patient for the procedure, and encourage her to lie in a lateral recumbent position.
- Inform the patient that she'll feel fluid flowing out of her vagina during the procedure.
- Make sure that the solution for infusion is warmed to the patient's body temperature to avoid chilling.
- Obtain a baseline fetal heart rate (FHR) tracing, and monitor the FHR continuously for changes from the baseline.

PROCEDURE

- The health care provider ruptures the membranes if they haven't ruptured spontaneously.
- The health care provider inserts a sterile pressure catheter through the cervix into the uterus.
- The catheter is attached via I.V. tubing to a warmed isotonic solution.
- The fluid is administered rapidly; usually 500 ml is given initially, after which the flow rate is titrated according to the FHR.
- Assist with infusion, and adjust the flow rate, as ordered, to maintain an FHR pattern demonstrating no variable decelerations.

POSTPROCEDURE CARE

■ Continuously monitor the FHR and uterine contractions.
■ Assess temperature every hour to detect infection.
■ Monitor the patient for a continuous flow of fluid from the vagina.
■ Provide comfort measures, including frequent bed linen changes.

ALERT *Notify the health care provider if the fluid suddenly stops — an indication that the fetal head is engaged and that fluid is collecting in the uterus, which could lead to hydramnios and possible uterine rupture.*

Amniotomy

DESCRIPTION

■ Artificial rupture of the amniotic sac
■ Allows the fetal head to contact the cervix more directly, thus increasing the efficiency of contractions
■ Associated risks:
  – Umbilical cord prolapse
  – Maternal infection
  – Possible abruptio placentae if the patient has hydramnios
■ Uterine collapse due to the draining fluid; decreasing area of placental attachment
■ Placenta no longer fitting the implantation site, decreasing the surface area of fetal oxygenation

PURPOSE

■ Means of augmenting or inducing labor
■ Allows internal fetal monitoring and access for fetal blood sampling

PATIENT PREPARATION

■ Before an amniotomy is done, the following factors must be present:
  – The fetus must be in the vertex position with the fetal head at −2 station or lower and a Bishop score of at least 8.
  – The patient's cervix must be dilated at least 3 cm.
■ Explain the rationale for the procedure.
■ Inform the patient that the procedure will be virtually painless (there are no nerve endings in the membranes).

DEALING WITH UMBILICAL CORD PROLAPSE

Umbilical cord prolapse is an emergency. Immediate action must be taken to relieve the pressure and to prevent fetal anoxia and fetal distress. Here are some options:
- Insert a gloved hand into the vagina, and gently push the fetal presenting part away from the cord.
- Place the patient in the Trendelenburg position to tilt the presenting part backward into the pelvis and relieve pressure on the cord.
- Administer oxygen by face mask to improve oxygen flow to the fetus.
    If the cord has prolapsed to the point that it's visible outside the vagina, don't attempt to push it back in. This can add to the compression and may cause kinking. Cover the exposed portion with a compress soaked with sterile saline solution to prevent drying, which could result in atrophy of the umbilical vessels.

- Institute continuous fetal monitoring.

PROCEDURE

- Place the patient in the dorsal recumbent position.
- Clean the perineum with soap and water or gauze pads moistened with an antiseptic agent.
- Place a linen-saver pad under the patient's buttocks.
- The health care provider inserts a hemostat or Amniohook (a long thin instrument similar to a crochet hook) into the vagina.
- Assist with applying pressure to the uterine fundus, if ordered, as the health care provider inserts the device.
- The health care provider tears or punctures the membranes.
- If the tear or puncture has been performed properly, the amniotic fluid will gush out.

POSTPROCEDURE CARE

- Watch for the flow of amniotic fluid, which should be clear.
- Report bloody or meconium-stained fluid, and continue close monitoring of the patient and fetus.
- Monitor the fetal heart rate continuously to detect indications of fetal distress or evidence of umbilical cord prolapse. (See *Dealing with umbilical cord prolapse.*)

ALERT *Umbilical cord prolapse is a life-threatening compli-cation of amniotomy. It's an emergency that requires im-mediate cesarean birth to prevent fetal death. Cord prolapse can lead to cord compression as the fetal presenting part presses the cord against the pelvic brim. Immediate action is crucial.*

- Assess maternal temperature every 2 hours.
- Assist the patient in progressing through labor.
- Prepare for delivery of the fetus.

Cerclage

DESCRIPTION

- Surgical procedure used to treat cervical insufficiency involving the use of a heavy suture placed at the internal cervical os
- May be done as an outpatient procedure, during a short 1- to 2-day hospitalization, or as an emergency procedure requiring hospitalization for approximately 5 days
- Usually performed during the late first trimester or early second trimester
- May be removed at approximately 37 weeks' gestation or kept in place with plans for cesarean delivery

PURPOSE

- Treatment of cervical insufficiency to help keep the cervix closed until term or until the patient goes into labor, for patients who have experi-enced previous pregnancy losses

PATIENT PREPARATION

- Explain the procedure and the rationale for its use.
- Ensure that the patient has followed preoperative instructions as indi-cated (if being performed on an outpatient basis).
- Assess for conditions that would contraindicate the procedure, includ-ing intra-amniotic infection, fetal death, fetal anomaly, vaginal bleed-ing, or premature rupture of membranes.
- If an emergency cerclage is being performed, expect to administer tocolytics, broad-spectrum antibiotics, and anti-inflammatory agents preoperatively.

PROCEDURE

- The patient receives regional anesthesia.
- The health care provider uses a suture or band to close the cervix using a vaginal approach.
- In a McDonald cerclage, the health care provider uses sutures placed horizontally and vertically high up on the cervix to pull it tightly together.
- In Shirodkar's procedure, the health care provider uses a submucosal band applied at the level of the internal cervical os.

POSTPROCEDURE CARE

- Maintain the patient on bed rest as ordered.
- Assess for evidence of uterine contractions and rupture of membranes.
- Monitor vital signs, especially temperature.
- Assess for signs and symptoms of infection.
- Provide emotional support to the patient, who has most likely experienced several pregnancy losses.
- Teach the patient how to monitor uterine contractions.
- Instruct the patient in signs and symptoms of preterm labor and the need to notify her health care provider immediately.
- Review activity restrictions or limitations.
- Anticipate the need for home uterine monitoring and home health care follow-up.

Cesarean birth

DESCRIPTION

- One of the oldest surgical procedures known
- May be performed as a planned surgery or as an emergency procedure when vaginal birth isn't possible (see *Cesarean delivery factors*)
- Can result in systemic effects, including thrombophlebitis from interference in the body's natural stress response as well as alterations in body defenses, circulatory function, organ function, self-image, and self-esteem
- Considered more hazardous than vaginal birth; performed only when the health and safety of the patient or fetus are in jeopardy
- Maternal complications: respiratory tract infection, wound dehiscence,

CESAREAN DELIVERY FACTORS

Cesarean delivery may be planned or performed as an emergency procedure. Factors that lead to cesarean birth may be maternal, placental, or fetal.

Maternal
- Cephalopelvic disproportion
- Active genital herpes or papilloma
- Previous cesarean birth by classic incision
- Disabling conditions, such as severe pregnancy-induced hypertension and heart disease, that prevent pushing to accomplish the pelvic division of labor

Placental
- Placenta previa
- Premature separation of the placenta

Fetal
- Transverse fetal lie
- Extremely low fetal size
- Fetal distress
- Compound conditions such as macrosomic fetus in a breech lie

thromboembolism, paralytic ileus, hemorrhage, genitourinary tract infection, and bowel, bladder, or uterine injury
- Generally contraindicated when there's a documented dead fetus (in this situation, labor can be induced to avoid an unnecessary surgical procedure)
- Also called *cesarean section* or *cesarean delivery*

PURPOSE

- Cesarean birth is indicated when labor or vaginal birth carries an unacceptable risk for the patient or fetus, including:
  - cephalopelvic disproportion
  - uterine dysfunction
  - malposition or malpresentation
  - previous uterine surgery
  - complete or partial placenta previa
  - preexisting medical condition (for example, diabetes or cardiac disease)

- prolapsed umbilical cord
- fetal distress, including a living fetus with a prolapsed cord, fetal hypoxia, abnormal fetal heart rate patterns, an unfavorable intrauterine environment (for example, because of infection), and moderate to severe Rh isoimmunization.

■ It may also be necessary if induction is contraindicated or difficult or if advanced labor increases the risk of morbidity and mortality.

■ Unless indicated by an emergency condition, the procedure is considered elective because the patient and her health care provider choose the date on which it will be performed based on the due date and the maturity of the fetus.

■ Cesarean delivery is usually planned when the patient has had a previous cesarean birth.

■ Vaginal birth after cesarean birth isn't recommended.

PATIENT PREPARATION

■ Assess maternal and fetal status frequently until delivery, as facility policy directs.

■ If ordered, make sure that an ultrasound has been obtained. The health care provider may have ordered the test to determine fetal position.

■ Explain cesarean delivery to the patient and her family, and answer any questions they may have.

■ Provide reassurance and emotional support to help improve the patient's self-esteem. Remember that a cesarean birth is commonly performed after hours of labor, resulting in an exhausted patient. Be brief but clear, and stress the essential points about the procedure.

■ For a scheduled cesarean birth, discuss the procedure with the patient and her family and provide preoperative teaching.

■ Observe the patient for signs of imminent delivery.

■ Demonstrate use of the incentive spirometer, and have the patient practice deep breathing. Review splinting measures to decrease incisional pain with deep breathing and coughing.

■ Restrict food and fluids after midnight if a general anesthetic is ordered to prevent aspiration of vomitus.

■ Prepare the patient's abdominal area, according to facility policy.

■ Make sure the patient's bladder is empty, use an indwelling urinary catheter as ordered, and check for flow and patency. Tell the patient that the catheter may remain in place for 24 hours or longer.

- Administer ordered preoperative medication.
- Give the patient an antacid, if ordered.
- Start an I.V. infusion for fluid replacement therapy using the patient's nondominant hand, if required. Use an 18G or larger catheter to allow blood administration through the I.V. line, if needed.
- Make sure the health care provider has ordered typing and crossmatching of the patient's blood and that 2 units of blood are available.
- Prepare the patient and family for what they might see. This can help avert too much shock or surprise as well as promote open discussion about how much they would like to see or not see.

PROCEDURE

- The patient receives general or regional anesthesia, depending on the extent of maternal or fetal distress.
- The patient is positioned on the operating table. A towel may be placed under her left hip to help relocate abdominal contents so that they're up and away from the surgical field. This can also assist in lifting the uterus off the vena cava, promoting better circulation to the fetus as well as maternal blood return.
- A metal screen or some other type of shielding may be placed at the patient's shoulder level and covered with a sterile drape.
- A family member, if present, is usually positioned at the patient's head.
- The incision area on the patient's abdomen is then scrubbed, and drapes are placed around the area of incision so that only a small area of skin is left exposed.
- The health care provider makes an incision through the skin and subcutaneous tissue, which is held open with retractors. (See *Types of cesarean incisions,* page 154.)
- Next, the uterus is incised and the neonate's head is delivered manually or with the use of forceps.
- The neonate's mouth and nose are suctioned, as done with a vaginal delivery.
- The remainder of the neonate's body is delivered followed by manual removal of the placenta and membranes.
- Oxytocin infusion is initiated to assist in uterine contraction.
- The neonate's umbilical cord is cut.
- The health care provider inspects the surgical area and then sutures the uterus, subcutaneous tissue, and skin.

TYPES OF CESAREAN INCISIONS

The type of incision chosen for cesarean delivery depends on the presentation of the fetus and the speed with which the procedure can be performed. In general, there are two types of cesarean incisions: classic and transverse, or low segment.

Transverse incision

The transverse incision, also known as the *bikini* or *low-segment incision,* is the preferred and most common incision.

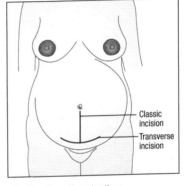

Classic incision

Transverse incision

- The incidence of peritonitis and postoperative adhesions is decreased with this type of incision.
- Blood loss is minimal.
- To decrease the risk of rupture during future labors, this incision is made in the lower portion of the uterus, which is minimally active with contractions.
- Vaginal birth after cesarean delivery is possible with this incision.

Classic incision

The classic, or vertical, incision is used when adhesions from previous cesarean delivery exist, when the fetus is in a transverse lie, or when the placenta is anteriorly implanted.

- The incision is made through the abdomen, high on the uterus.
- This type of incision may be used for patients with placenta previa because the incision can be made without cutting the placenta.
- The chances of vaginal birth after cesarean birth with this type of incision are low because of the incision's location in the major active contracting portion of the uterus.

POSTPROCEDURE CARE

- As soon as possible, allow the patient to see, touch, and hold her neonate, either in the delivery room or after she recovers from the general anesthetic. Contact with the neonate promotes bonding.
- Check the perineal pad and abdominal dressing on the incision every

15 minutes for 1 hour, then every half hour for 4 hours, every hour for 4 hours, and finally every 4 hours for 24 hours.

- Perform fundal checks at the same intervals. Gently assess the fundus.
- Check the dressing frequently for bleeding, and report it immediately. Be sure to keep the incision clean and dry.
- Monitor vital signs every 5 minutes until stable. Then check vital signs when you evaluate perineal and abdominal drainage.
- The physician may order oxytocin mixed in with the first 1,000 to 2,000 ml of I.V. fluids infused to promote uterine contraction and decrease the risk of hemorrhage. Make sure the I.V. is patent, and monitor the patient carefully for effects of the medication.
- Monitor intake and output as ordered. Expect the patient to receive I.V. fluids for 24 to 48 hours.
- Make sure that the catheter is patent and that urine flow is adequate. When the catheter is removed, make sure that the patient can void without difficulty and that urine color and amount are adequate.
- Maintain a patent airway for the patient and the neonate.
- Encourage the patient to cough and deep-breathe and to use the incentive spirometer to promote adequate respiratory function.
- If a general anesthetic was used, remain with the patient until she's responsive; if a regional anesthetic was used, monitor the return of sensation to the legs.
- Help the patient to turn from side to side every 1 to 2 hours.
- Administer pain medication as ordered, and provide comfort measures for breast engorgement as appropriate.
- If ordered, show the patient how to administer patient-controlled analgesia.
- If the patient wants to breast-feed, offer encouragement and help.
- Recognize afterpains in multiparas, and monitor the effects of pain medication. Timing of administration of pain medication and breast-feeding may need to be coordinated so that the neonate won't receive as much of the sedating effect.
- Promote early ambulation to prevent cardiovascular and pulmonary complications.

ALERT *Assist the patient with getting out of bed the first time to prevent injury that may occur because of orthostatic hypotension. Also, stay alert for an increase in lochia when she moves from a supine to an upright position.*

- Instruct the patient to immediately report hemorrhage, chest or leg

pain (possible thrombosis), dyspnea, or separation of the wound's edges.
- Tell her to also report signs and symptoms of infection, such as fever, difficulty urinating, and flank pain.
- Remind the patient to keep her follow-up appointment.

Episiotomy

DESCRIPTION

- A surgical incision of the perineum used to enlarge the vaginal outlet
- Classified by the site and direction of the incision (see *Types of episiotomy incisions*)
- Advantages:
  - Prevents tearing (laceration) of the perineum
  - Can be repaired more easily than a tear and heals faster
  - Enlarges the vaginal outlet to facilitate manipulation or the use of forceps or vacuum extraction
- Disadvantages:
  - Interference with maternal-neonatal bonding if discomfort is severe
  - Risk of infection
  - Hesitancy by the patient to void or have a bowel movement because of discomfort

PURPOSE

- Used to prevent the perineum from tearing, which can occur with birth
- Helps to release the pressure on the fetal head that accompanies preterm birth

PATIENT PREPARATION

- Explain the procedure and its rationale to the patient and her family.
- Inform the patient that she may receive a local anesthetic.
- Tell the patient that she may experience some discomfort in the area after the procedure.

PROCEDURE

- A pudendal nerve block may be administered.

TYPES OF EPISIOTOMY INCISIONS

An episiotomy incision may be midline or mediolateral, as shown below.

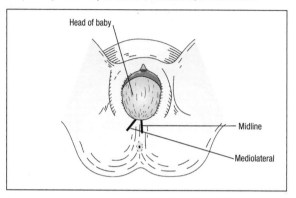

Midline episiotomy
- Involves an incision that's made in the middle of the perineum
- Advantageous because it's associated with easier healing, decreased blood loss, and decreased postpartum discomfort

Mediolateral episiotomy
- Involves an incision begun at the midline and then angled to one side away from the rectum (can be right or left)
- Advantageous because of the decreased risk of rectal mucosa tears

- Using a blunt-tipped scissor, the health care provider makes an incision in the midline of the perineum or makes an incision beginning at the midline and angled laterally away from the rectum on either the right or left side.
- After delivery of the neonate and placenta, the episiotomy is sutured closed.

POSTPROCEDURE CARE

- Provide postpartum care as usual.
- Apply ice packs to the perineum for the first 24 hours to help reduce swelling and promote comfort.

- Carefully inspect the episiotomy when performing perineal checks. Notify the health care provider of any increased redness, swelling, drainage, or hematoma formation.
- Reinforce the need for frequent perineal care.
- Assist with pain management, including the use of oral analgesics and topical medications; instruct the patient in how to use topical medications.
- After the first 24 hours, instruct the patient in using a sitz bath and explain that the baths will promote comfort, reduce edema, and promote healing.

Forceps delivery

DESCRIPTION

- Used to assist with delivery and to relieve fetal head compression
- Two types: Low-forceps or midforceps
- Risks:
  - Perinatal morbidity and mortality (midforceps delivery)
  - Neonatal birth trauma and depression
  - Perineal lacerations
  - Postpartum hemorrhage
  - Bladder injury

PURPOSE

- Assists with delivery when adverse fetal and maternal conditions exist
- Aids in relieving fetal head compression

PATIENT PREPARATION

- Explain the procedure and its rationale to the patient and her family.
- Advise the patient that she may receive a local anesthetic to relax the pelvic area and to reduce pain.
- Inform the patient that she'll be instructed when and when not to push.
- Monitor fetal heart rate (FHR) patterns before the forceps are applied.

■ Ensure that the following are present: ruptured membranes, fully dilated cervix, empty bladder, and absence of cephalopelvic disproportion.

PROCEDURE

■ Assist with administration of an anesthetic, if indicated.
■ Monitor the patient and notify the health care provider when a contraction begins; instruct the patient not to push at this time.
■ The health care provider slides one blade of the forceps into the patient's vagina on one side of the fetus's head.
■ Next, he slides the other blade on the opposite side of the fetus's head.
■ He then brings the shaft of each blade together, forming a handle.
■ After insertion of the forceps, assess the FHR again to ensure that the cord isn't being compressed by the forceps.
■ During a contraction, the health care provider applies traction to aid in moving the fetus; the patient is now instructed to push.
■ A low-forceps (outlet) delivery is performed when the fetus's head reaches the perineum; typically, the fetal head is at –2 station or more.
■ A midforceps delivery is performed when the fetal head is engaged but is at less than –2 station; because of the increased risk of birth trauma, this type of delivery is rarely done.

POSTPROCEDURE CARE

■ Provide postpartum care as usual.
■ Assess the patient's perineal area and cervix; report any signs of lacerations.
■ Encourage the patient to void soon after birth.

ALERT *Bladder injury is possible when forceps are used. Therefore, be sure to document the time and amount of first voiding to ensure adequate bladder function. If the patient is unable to void within 6 to 8 hours after birth, notify the health care provider.*

■ Warn the mother that she may notice a reddened area or some bruising on the neonate's cheeks from the application of the forceps. Inform her that this will fade in 1 to 2 days.
■ Assess the neonate for possible facial palsy or subdural hematoma from application of the forceps.

Labor induction and augmentation

DESCRIPTION

- *Induction* is artificial initiation of labor.
- *Augmentation* is assisting labor that started spontaneously.
- For induction, the fetus must be mature, in longitudinal lie, engaged, and in cephalopelvic proportion (the fetal head can pass through the pelvis).
- The patient must have a ripe cervix (soft and supple to the touch rather than firm), which allows for cervical effacement, dilation, and effective coordination of contractions. (See *Evaluating cervical readiness*, page 24.)
- Several methods may be used to induce labor: amniotomy, prostaglandin administration, or oxytocin administration.
- Amniotomy involves the artificial rupturing of membranes with a sterile instrument; under favorable conditions, about 80% of patients enter labor within 24 hours. (See "Amniotomy," page 147.)
- Induction using prostaglandin (prostaglandin E_2 such as dinoprostone [Cervidil, Prepidil, or Prostin E_2]) involves the intracervical or intravaginal insertion of prostaglandin gel to soften (ripen) the cervix; agents initiate the breakdown of the collagen that keeps the cervix tightly closed.
- Induction with oxytocin involves the administration of I.V. oxytocin (Pitocin) as an infusion to augment or stimulate uterine contractions.
- Labor induction and augmentation should be done cautiously in women age 35 and older and in those with grand parity or uterine scars.
- It shouldn't be done if:
  - vaginal birth is too risky
  - stimulation of the uterus increases the risk of such complications as placenta previa, abruptio placentae, uterine rupture, and decreased fetal blood supply caused by the increased intensity or duration of contractions
  - multiple pregnancy is involved
  - the patient has an active genital herpes infection
  - evidence of fetal distress exists
  - the fetus is in an unusual presentation (such as a footling breech presentation)
  - the uterus is unusually large (which increases the risk of uterine rupture).

PURPOSE

- Induction used to safeguard the health of the mother or fetus when pregnancy is considered high risk or when such medical conditions as preeclampsia, eclampsia, severe hypertension, diabetes, Rh sensitization, prolonged rupture of membranes (over 24 hours), and a postmature fetus (a fetus that's 42 weeks' gestation or older) occur
- Augmentation of labor used if the contractions are too weak or infrequent to be effective

PATIENT PREPARATION

- Explain the procedure to be used and the reason for its use.
- Review the possible risks and benefits to the patient and the fetus.
- Instruct the patient about signs and symptoms that should be reported immediately.
- Explain the necessary assessments and monitoring activities to be performed.
- Inform the patient of the need to lie flat after the application of prostaglandin E_2 to prevent expulsion of the medication.
- Determine whether the patient has received a prostaglandin ripening agent.

ALERT *Oxytocin induction can be started 6 to 12 hours after the last application of prostaglandin. If oxytocin is started earlier, hyperstimulation of the uterus may occur.*

PROCEDURE

Amniotomy
See discussion on page 147.

Prostaglandin for cervical ripening
- Prostaglandin gel is applied to the interior surface of the cervix by a catheter or suppository, to the external surface of the cervix by applying it to a diaphragm and then placing the diaphragm against the cervix, or by vaginal insertion.
- Additional doses may be applied every 6 hours; however, two or three doses are usually enough to cause ripening.

Oxytocin infusion
- Start a primary I.V. line.

■ Prepare the oxytocin infusion; insert the tubing of the administration set through the infusion pump, and set the drip rate to administer the oxytocin at a starting infusion rate of 0.5 to 1.0 milliunits/minute.

ALERT *The maximum dosage of oxytocin is 20 to 40 milliunits/minute. Typically, the recommended labor-starting dosage is 10 units of oxytocin in 100 ml of isotonic solution to run at 0.5 to 1.0 milliunits/minute, with the maximum dosage being 20 to 40 mU.*

■ Piggyback the oxytocin solution to the primary I.V. line.
■ Continuously monitor uterine contractions and fetal heart rate (FHR) patterns. If a problem occurs, such as decelerations of the FHR or fetal distress, stop the piggyback infusion immediately and resume the primary line.
■ Increase the oxytocin dosage as ordered — but never increase the dose more than 2 milliunits/minute once every 30 to 60 minutes. Typically, the dosage continues at a rate that maintains activity closest to normal labor.

POSTPROCEDURE CARE

■ Help the patient participate in the labor process as much as possible.
■ Assess the patient's progress through labor.

Amniotomy
See discussion on page 147.

Prostaglandin for cervical ripening
■ Carefully monitor the patient's uterine activity.
■ If uterine hyperstimulation occurs or if labor begins, expect the prostaglandin agent to be removed.

ALERT *A prostaglandin cervical-ripening product must be removed from the cervix before oxytocin administration because prostaglandin potentiates the effect of oxytocin. Prostaglandin must also be removed before amniotomy. Use this drug with caution in women with asthma, glaucoma, or renal or cardiac disease.*

■ Monitor the patient for adverse effects of prostaglandin application, including headache, vomiting, fever, diarrhea, and hypertension.
■ Monitor the FHR continuously for at least 30 minutes after each application and for up to 2 hours after vaginal insertion.

COMPLICATIONS OF OXYTOCIN ADMINISTRATION

Oxytocin can cause uterine hyperstim-ulation. This, in turn, may progress to tetanic contractions, which last longer than 2 minutes. Signs of hyperstimu-lation include contractions less than 2 minutes apart and lasting 90 seconds or longer, uterine pressure that does-n't return to baseline between con-tractions, and intrauterine pressure that rises to more than 75 mm Hg.

Additional potential complications
Other potential complications include fetal distress, abruptio placentae, and uterine rupture. In addition, watch for signs of oxytocin hypersensitivity such as elevated blood pressure. Rarely, oxytocin leads to maternal seizures or coma from water intoxication.

Contraindications
Contraindications to administering oxytocin include placenta previa, diag-nosed cephalopelvic disproportion, fetal distress, prior classic uterine incision or uterine surgery, and active genital herpes. Oxytocin should be administered cautiously to a patient who has an overdistended uterus or a history of cervical surgery, uterine surgery, or grand multiparity.

■ Advise the patient to remain supine after application to prevent leak-age of the medication.

Oxytocin infusion
■ Before each increase, be sure to assess contractions, maternal vital signs, and the FHR.

ALERT When using an external fetal monitor, the uterine activity strip or grid should show contractions occurring every 2 to 3 minutes. The contractions should last for about 60 seconds and be followed by uterine relaxation. If using an inter-nal fetal monitor, look for an optimal baseline value ranging from 5 to 15 mm Hg. The goal is to verify uterine relaxation between contractions.

■ Assist with comfort measures, such as repositioning the patient on her other side, as needed.
■ Continue assessing maternal and fetal responses to the oxytocin.

ALERT Always administer oxytocin solution as a piggy-back to the primary I.V. line using an infusion pump; if a problem occurs, such as decelerations of the FHR or fetal distress, the piggyback infusion can be stopped immediately and the pri-

mary line resumed. Stop the infusion immediately if fetal distress or tetanic contractions occur.

■ Review the infusion rate to prevent uterine hyperstimulation. To manage hyperstimulation, discontinue the infusion and administer oxygen. (See *Complications of oxytocin administration,* page 163.)

■ To reduce uterine irritability, use measures to increase uterine blood flow: change the patient's position, and increase the infusion rate of the primary I.V. line. After hyperstimulation resolves, resume the oxytocin infusion per facility policy.

Tocolytic therapy
DESCRIPTION

■ Use of medications to suppress uterine activity
■ May include magnesium sulfate, terbutaline (Brethine), nifedipine (Procardia), or indomethacin (Indocin) (see *Tocolytic drugs*)
■ Contraindications: gestation less than 20 weeks, cervical dilation

---

TOCOLYTIC DRUGS

This chart highlights the major drugs used to halt uterine contractions.

Drug	Indications
Terbutaline (Brethine)	Beta$_2$ receptor stimulator that causes smooth-muscle relaxation
Magnesium sulfate	Central nervous system (CNS) depressant that prevents reflux of calcium into the myometrial cells, thereby keeping the uterus relaxed
	Prostaglandin synthesis inhibitor; typically not used after 32 weeks' gestation, to avoid premature closure of the ductus arteriosus
Indomethacin (Indocin)	Nonsteroidal anti-inflammatory that decreases production of prostaglandins, which are lipid compounds associated with the initiation of labor
Nifedipine (Procardia)	Calcium channel blocker that decreases the production of calcium, a substance associated with the initiation of labor

greater than 4 cm, ruptured membranes, and cervical effacement greater than 50%

PURPOSE

- To stop preterm labor contractions or to prevent preterm labor

PATIENT PREPARATION

- Assess baseline uterine contractions and fetal heart rate (FHR) patterns.
- Explain the drug therapy ordered, including the route used and possible adverse effects.
- Start an I.V. line for the patient who will receive magnesium sulfate or terbutaline I.V.
- Obtain laboratory studies, including complete blood count, hemoglobin level, hematocrit, and serum electrolyte levels.
- Obtain a baseline electrocardiogram and cultures of urine, the vagina, and the cervix, as ordered.

Effects on the mother	Effects on the fetus	Antidote
Tachycardia, diarrhea, nervousness and tremors, nausea and vomiting, headache, hyperglycemia or hypoglycemia, hypokalemia, and pulmonary edema	Tachycardia, hypoxia, hypoglycemia, and hypocalcemia	Propranolol (Inderal)
Drowsiness, flushing, warmth, nausea, headache, slurred speech, and blurred vision (toxicity is manifested by CNS depression, respirations less than 12 breaths/minute, hyporeflexia, oliguria, cardiac arrhythmias, and cardiac arrest)	Hypotonia and bradycardia	Calcium gluconate
Nausea, vomiting, and dyspepsia; additive CNS effects if given with magnesium sulfate	Premature closure of ductus arteriosus	None; discontinuation of drug necessary
Headache, flushing; additive CNS effects if given with magnesium sulfate	Minimal	None; discontinuation of drug necessary

- Closely observe the patient who's in preterm labor for signs of fetal or maternal distress, and provide comprehensive supportive care.
- Provide guidance about the hospital stay, the potential for delivery of a preterm neonate, and the possible need for neonatal intensive care.
- Encourage the patient to assume a side-lying position to maximize placental blood flow and relieve pressure on the cervix.
- During attempts to suppress preterm labor, make sure the patient maintains bed rest; provide appropriate diversionary activities.

PROCEDURE

- Administer the tocolytic agent as ordered.
- Give nifedipine and indomethacin orally; give magnesium sulfate as an I.V. infusion piggybacked into a primary line; give terbutaline subcutaneously or as an I.V. infusion piggybacked into a primary line.

POSTPROCEDURE CARE

- Continue administration of tocolytic therapy as ordered.
- Monitor blood pressure, pulse rate, respirations, FHR, and uterine contraction pattern when administering a beta-adrenergic stimulant.
- Minimize adverse reactions by keeping the patient in a side-lying position as much as possible to ensure adequate placental perfusion.

> **ALERT** *Monitor the status of contractions, notifying the health care provider if the patient experiences more than four contractions per hour. If the mother's pulse rises above 120 beats/minute, if her systolic blood pressure drops below 90 mm Hg, or if the fetus's heart rate rises above 180 beats/minute or drops below 110 beats/minute, notify the health care provider.*

- Administer fluids, as ordered, to ensure adequate hydration; monitor intake and output to prevent fluid overload.
- Frequently assess deep tendon reflexes when administering magnesium sulfate. (See *Safety with magnesium.*)
- Prepare the patient for possible delivery if therapy is unsuccessful; if preterm labor continues, expect to administer corticosteroids to promote lung maturity in the fetus.

SAFETY WITH MAGNESIUM

Use caution when administering I.V. magnesium therapy by following these guidelines.

- Always administer the drug as a piggyback infusion so that if the patient develops signs and symptoms of toxicity, the drug can be discontinued immediately.
- Obtain a baseline serum magnesium level before initiating therapy, and monitor frequently thereafter.
- Keep in mind that to be effective as an anticonvulsant, serum magnesium levels should be between 5 and 8 mg/dl. Levels above 8 mg/dl indicate toxicity and place the patient at risk for respiratory depression, cardiac arrhythmias, and cardiac arrest.
- Assess the patient's deep tendon reflexes. Ideally, this should be the patellar reflex. However, if the patient has received epidural anesthesia, test the biceps or triceps reflex. Diminished or hypoactive reflexes suggest magnesium toxicity.
- Assess for ankle clonus by rapidly dorsiflexing the patient's ankle three times in succession and then remove your hand, observing foot movement. If no further motion is noted, ankle clonus is absent; if the foot continues to move voluntarily, clonus is present. Moderate (three to five) or severe (six or more) movements may suggest magnesium toxicity.
- Have calcium gluconate readily available at the patient's bedside. Anticipate administering this antidote for magnesium toxicity.

- If labor isn't stopped and a preterm neonate is delivered, monitor the neonate for signs of magnesium toxicity, including neuromuscular and respiratory depression.
- If labor is suppressed, begin discharge teaching with the patient and her family about tocolytic therapy at home; anticipate referral for home care follow-up.
- Instruct the patient about drug dosage, frequency, route, and possible adverse effects.
- Teach the patient how to monitor contraction pattern, pulse rate, and fetal movement.
- Teach the patient the signs and symptoms of true labor.
- Review activity restrictions; discuss danger signs about which to notify the health care provider.

Vacuum extraction

DESCRIPTION

- An alternative to forceps delivery
- Lower incidence of vaginal, cervical, and third- and fourth-degree lacerations, less maternal discomfort (because the cup doesn't occupy additional space in the birth canal and less anesthesia is necessary than that required for forceps delivery)
- Associated with a marked caput succedaneum of the neonate's head, lasting as long as 7 days after birth
- Risks: tentorial tears from extreme pressure; renewed bleeding from the scalp following fetal blood sampling
- Problematic in a preterm neonate due to extreme softness of skull
- Also called *vacuum-assisted birth*

PURPOSE

- To facilitate descent of the fetal head
- To assist in shortening the second stage of labor

PATIENT PREPARATION

- Explain the procedure and its rationale to the patient and her family.
- Monitor uterine contractions and fetal heart rate frequently.
- Inform the patient that the pressure and traction will be applied during contractions; encourage her to push when directed.
- Assess the patient for possible contraindications for the procedure, including true cephalopelvic disproportion, nonvertex presentations, maternal or suspected fetal coagulation problems, hydrocephalus (known or suspected), and trauma to the fetal scalp.
- Inform the patient and her family that the neonate's head may be temporarily misshapen from application of the suction.
- Encourage the patient to participate in the labor process as much as possible.

PROCEDURE

- A plastic vacuum cup connected to a suction source via tubing is applied to the fetal head over the sagittal suture, 3 cm above the posterior fontanel. (See *Vacuum extraction*.)

- Negative pressure of approximately 50 to 60 mm Hg is exerted, causing air beneath the cup to be removed.
- The cup adheres tightly to the fetal head.
- In conjunction with contractions, the health care provider applies traction.
- With each contraction, traction is applied until the fetus's head emerges from the birth canal.
- After the head has emerged from the birth canal, the vacuum cup is removed.

POSTPROCEDURE CARE

- Provide postpartum care as usual.
- Inspect the neonate's head for evidence of caput succedaneum, which is a common result of using the vacuum cup.
- Assess the neonate for possible complications, such as cephalohematoma, and for signs of trauma and infection.
- Monitor the neonate for signs of listlessness or poor sucking, which may indicate cerebral irritation.
- Inform the patient and her family that the neonate's head will resume its normal shape in about 1 week.
- Inform neonatal caregivers and personnel that vacuum extraction was used.

VACUUM EXTRACTION

With vacuum extraction, a suction cup is applied to the fetal head at the posterior fontanel. Negative pressure via suction is used, and traction is applied to achieve delivery.

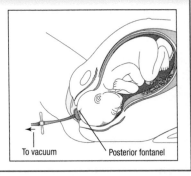

To vacuum   Posterior fontanel

Procedures

Part three

Apgar scoring

DESCRIPTION

- Quantification of neonate's status based on observations of neonate's appearance and behavior
- Developed by anesthesiologist Dr. Virginia Apgar in 1952
- Evaluation of neonatal heart rate, respiratory effort, muscle tone, reflex irritability, and color

EQUIPMENT

Stethoscope ◆ gloves

ESSENTIAL STEPS

- Perform evaluation of each category at 1 minute after birth and again at 5 minutes after birth.
- Score each category as 0, 1, or 2.
- Obtain the final Apgar score by adding the scores for each category; the maximum score is 10.

Heart rate

- Assess heart rate first.
- If the umbilical cord still pulsates, palpate the neonate's heart rate by placing your fingertips at the junction of the umbilical cord and the skin.

> **ALERT** *The neonate's cord stump continues to pulsate for several hours and is a good, easy place (next to the abdomen) to check heart rate. When palpating at the cord stump, be sure to wear gloves.*

- Alternatively, place two fingers or a stethoscope over the neonate's chest at the fifth intercostal space to obtain an apical pulse.
- Count the heart rate for 1 full minute.

Respiratory effort

- Assess the neonate's cry, noting its volume and vigor.

- Auscultate his lungs, using a stethoscope.
- Assess his respirations for depth and regularity.

  ALERT *If the neonate exhibits abnormal respiratory responses, begin neonatal resuscitation according to the guidelines of the American Heart Association and the American Academy of Pediatrics. Then use the Apgar score to judge the progress and success of resuscitation efforts.*

Muscle tone

- Determine muscle tone by evaluating the degree of flexion in the neonate's arms and legs and their resistance to straightening.
- Extend the limbs and observe their rapid return to flexion — the neonate's normal state.

Reflex irritability

- Evaluate the neonate's cry for presence, vigor, and pitch.

  ALERT *Be aware that initially the neonate may not cry. In this case, elicit a cry by flicking his soles. The usual response is a loud, angry cry. A high-pitched or shrill cry is abnormal.*

Color

- Observe skin color for cyanosis.
- Keep in mind that a neonate usually has a pink body with blue extremities (called *acrocyanosis*) due to decreased peripheral oxygenation caused by the transition from fetal to independent circulation.
- When assessing a nonwhite neonate, observe for color changes in the mucous membranes of the mouth, conjunctivae, lips, palms, and soles.

NURSING CONSIDERATIONS

- Remember that evaluation at 1 minute quickly indicates the neonate's initial adaptation to extrauterine life and whether resuscitation is necessary. The 5-minute score gives a more accurate picture of his overall status.
- Record the Apgar score. (See *Recording the Apgar score*, page 174.)

RECORDING THE APGAR SCORE

Use this chart to determine the neonatal Apgar score at 1-minute and 5-minute intervals after birth. For each category listed, assign a score of 0 to 2, as shown. A total score of 7 to 10 indicates that the neonate is in good condition; 4 to 6, fair condition (the neonate may have moderate central nervous system depression, muscle flaccidity, cyanosis, and poor respirations); 0 to 3, danger (the neonate needs immediate resuscitation as ordered).

Sign	Apgar score		
	0	1	2
Heart rate	Absent	Less than 100 beats/minute	More than 100 beats/minute
Respiratory effort	Absent	Slow, irregular	Good crying
Muscle tone	Flaccid	Some flexion and resistance to extension of extremities	Active motion
Reflex irritability	No response	Grimace or weak cry	Vigorous cry
Color	Pallor, cyanosis	Pink body, blue extremities	Completely pink

Cervical dilation and effacement assessment

DESCRIPTION

- Cervical dilation (the opening of the external cervical os): progresses from 0 to 10 cm
- Cervical effacement (cervical thinning and shortening): measured from 0% (palpable and thick) to 100% (fully indistinct and paper thin)
- Progress as labor advances, promoting delivery (See *Cervical dilation and effacement.*)

EQUIPMENT

Sterile gloves ◆ sterile water-soluble lubricant or sterile water ◆ mild soap and water or cleaning solution ◆ linen-saver pads ◆ antiseptic solution

CERVICAL DILATION AND EFFACEMENT

As labor advances, so do cervical dilation and effacement, which promote delivery. Cervical dilation — progressive widening of the cervical canal from the upper internal cervical os to the lower external cervical os — advances from 0 to 10 cm. As the cervical canal opens, resistance decreases. This further eases fetal descent.

At the same time, during effacement, the cervix shortens and its walls become thin. Full effacement obliterates the constrictive uterine neck to create a smooth, unobstructed passageway for the fetus.

NO DILATION OR EFFACEMENT

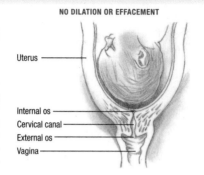

Uterus

Internal os
Cervical canal
External os
Vagina

FULL DILATION AND EFFACEMENT

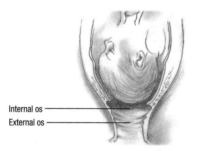

Internal os
External os

ESSENTIAL STEPS

- Prepare the patient for a vaginal examination.
- Confirm the patient's identity by using two patient identifiers according to facility policy.
- Explain the procedure to the patient and ask her to empty her bladder.
- Identify fetal presenting part and position using Leopold's maneuvers.
- Help the patient into a lithotomy position. Place a linen-saver pad under the patient's buttocks.
- Put on sterile gloves, and lubricate the index and middle fingers of your examining hand with sterile water or sterile water-soluble lubricant. If the membranes are ruptured, use an antiseptic solution.

- Ask the patient to relax by taking several deep breaths and slowly releasing the air.
- Insert lubricated fingers (palmar surface down) into the vagina. Keep your uninserted fingers flexed to avoid the rectum.
- Palpate the cervix, noting its consistency.

    ALERT *The cervix, on palpation, feels like a circular rim that surrounds a depression in the center. A firm cervix is similar in consistency to the tip of the nose; a soft cervix is similar in consistency to the earlobe.*

- Measure the extent of cervical dilation using the width of your fingertips as a guide.

    ALERT *The width of an index finger is approximately 1 cm; the width of a middle finger is approximately 1.5 cm. If both fingers can be inserted into the cervix, dilation is 2.5 to 3 cm. If the area permits insertion of your index and middle fingers twice across, cervical dilation is approximately 5 to 6 cm. If the area permits insertion of your index and middle fingers four times across, cervical dilation is 10 cm.*

- Estimate the percentage of cervical effacement by determining its thickness.

    ALERT *When the cervix is 0% effaced, it is approximately 2 to 2.5 cm thick; at 50% effacement, the cervix is about 1 cm thick; at 100% effacement, the cervix is paper thin.*

- Withdraw your fingers gently and wipe away any secretions, lubrication, or examining solution.
- Help the patient clean her perineum, and change the linen-saver pad as necessary.
- Reposition the patient comfortably.

NURSING CONSIDERATIONS

- Keep in mind that assessment for cervical dilation and effacement is commonly done during a vaginal examination in conjunction with assessing fetal station, presentation, and position.
- Adhere to standard precautions at all times.
- Don't perform the examination if bleeding is present or if there's evidence of the umbilical cord in the perineal area.
- Document your findings and how the patient tolerated the procedure.
- In early labor, assess cervical dilation and effacement in between con-

tractions; at the end of the first stage of labor, perform the assessment during a contraction to assist in determining fetal descent.
- After the membranes rupture, perform the assessment only when labor changes significantly, to minimize the risk of intrauterine infection.

External electronic fetal monitoring

DESCRIPTION

- Indirect, noninvasive procedure involving the use of two devices, an ultrasound transducer and a tocotransducer, placed on the mother's abdomen
- Aids in evaluating fetal well-being and uterine contractions during labor
- Devices held in place with an elastic stockinette or with plastic or soft straps
- Transmission of high-frequency sound waves aimed at the fetal heart via the ultrasound transducer
- Response to pressure exerted by uterine contractions via the tocotransducer with simultaneous recording of the duration and frequency of the contractions
- Resultant tracings of fetal heart rate (FHR) and uterine contraction data onto the same printout paper
- Used for most women, especially those with a high-risk pregnancy or oxytocin-induced labor

EQUIPMENT

Electronic fetal monitor and manufacturer's operating manual ◆ ultrasound transducer ◆ tocotransducer ◆ conductive gel ◆ transducer straps ◆ damp cloth ◆ printout paper

ESSENTIAL STEPS

- After reviewing the operating manual, prepare the machine for use.
- Label the monitoring strip with, or enter into the computer, the patient's identification number or birth date, her name, the date, maternal vital signs and position, the paper speed, and the number of the strip paper.

APPLYING EXTERNAL MONITORING DEVICES

To ensure clear tracings that define fetal status and labor progress, be sure to precisely position external monitoring devices. These devices include an ultra-sound transducer and a tocotransducer.

Fetal heart monitor
Palpate the uterus to locate the fetus's back and place the ultra-sound transducer, which reads the fetal heart rate, over the site where the fetal heartbeat sounds the loudest. Then tighten the belt. Use the fetal heart tracing on the monitor strip to confirm the transducer's position.

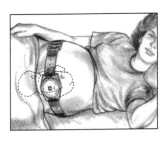

Tocotransducer
A tocotransducer records uterine motion during contractions. Place the tocotransducer over the uterine fundus where it contracts, either midline or slightly to one side. Place your hand on the fundus, and palpate a contraction to verify proper placement. Secure the tocotransducer's belt; then adjust the pen set so that the baseline values read between 5 and 15 mm Hg on the monitor strip.

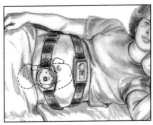

- Confirm the patient's identity by using two patient identifiers according to facility policy.
- Explain the procedure to the patient and make sure that she has signed a consent form, if required by the facility.
- Wash your hands and provide privacy.
- Assist the patient to the semi-Fowler or left-lateral position with her abdomen exposed, and palpate the abdomen to locate the fundus — the area of greatest muscle density in the uterus.
- Using transducer straps or a stockinette binder, secure the tocotransducer over the fundus. (See *Applying external monitoring devices.*)
- Adjust the pen set tracer controls so that the baseline values read between 5 and 15 mm Hg on the monitor strip or as indicated by the model.

- Apply conductive gel to the ultrasound transducer, and use Leopold's maneuvers to palpate the fetal back, through which fetal heart sounds resound most audibly.
- Start the monitor, and apply the ultrasound transducer directly over the site having the strongest heart sounds.
- Activate the control that begins the printout.
- Observe the tracings to identify the frequency and duration of uterine contractions, but palpate the uterus to determine intensity of contractions.
- Note the baseline FHR and assess periodic accelerations or decelerations from the baseline. Compare the FHR patterns with those of the uterine contractions.

NURSING CONSIDERATIONS

- Move the tocotransducer and the ultrasound transducer to accommodate changes in maternal or fetal position.
- Readjust both transducers every hour, and assess the patient's skin for reddened areas caused by the pressure of the monitoring device.
- Clean the ultrasound transducer periodically with a damp cloth to remove dried conduction gel, and apply fresh gel as necessary.
- If the patient reports discomfort in the position that provides the clearest signal, try to obtain a satisfactory 5- or 10-minute tracing with the patient in this position before assisting her to a more comfortable position.
- Number each fetal monitoring strip in sequence and label each printout sheet with the patient's identification number or birth date, name, date and time, and paper speed.
- Also record the time of vaginal exams, membrane rupture, drug administration, and maternal or fetal movements.
- Record the intensity of the uterine contractions and each movement or readjustment of the tocotransducer and ultrasound transducer.
- Continue to assess the patient and document any interventions necessary in correlation with the monitor printout strips.

Eye prophylaxis
DESCRIPTION

- Instillation of antibiotic ointment into the neonate's eyes for prevention of blindness and eye damage from conjunctivitis due to *Neisseria gonorrhoeae* and *Chlamydia*, which the neonate may have acquired from the mother during passage through the birth canal.

- Legally required in all 50 states
- Drug of choice: erythromycin ointment 0.5%

EQUIPMENT

Antibiotic ointment, usually single-dose ointment tube ◆ sterile gloves ◆ dry gauze pads

ESSENTIAL STEPS

- Obtain a prescribed ointment.
- Explain the procedure to the patient and family members (if present), informing them that the neonate will probably cry and that eye irritation may occur.
- Confirm the identity of the neonate using two patient identifiers according to facility policy.
- Wash your hands and put on gloves.
- Wipe the neonate's face with dry gauze.
- Shield the neonate's eyes from direct light and tilt his head slightly to the side of the intended treatment.
- Using your nondominant hand, gently raise the neonate's upper eyelid with your index finger and pull the lower eyelid down with your thumb.
- Using your dominant hand, instill a 1- to 2-cm ribbon of ointment along the lower conjunctival sac, from the inner canthus to the outer canthus.
- Close the neonate's eye to allow the ointment to be distributed across the conjunctiva.
- Repeat the steps with the other eye.

NURSING CONSIDERATIONS

- Use a single-dose ointment tube to prevent contamination and the spread of infection.
- Keep in mind that although the procedure may be administered in the birthing room, treatment can be delayed for up to 1 hour to allow initial parent-child bonding.
- Assess the neonate's eyes for chemical conjunctivitis evidenced by red-

ness, swelling, and drainage or discoloration of the skin around the
neonate's eyes.
- If chemical conjunctivitis or discoloration occurs, inform the parents
that these effects are temporary and will subside within a few days.
- Document the procedure appropriately on the birthing room record or
in the progress notes.

Fetal heart rate assessment

DESCRIPTION

- Noninvasive method of obtaining fetal heart rate (FHR) involving the
use of a Doppler ultrasound device or fetoscope
- FHR detectable at 12 weeks' gestation via Doppler ultrasound device
- FHR detectable at 16 to 20 weeks' via fetoscope
- Normal FHR ranging from 120 to 160 beats/minute
- Important source of information about fetal well-being

EQUIPMENT

Fetoscope or Doppler ultrasound device ◆ water-soluble lubricant ◆
watch with second hand ◆ bath blanket

ESSENTIAL STEPS

- Confirm the patient's identity by using two patient identifiers accord-
ing to facility policy.
- Explain the procedure to the patient.
- Wash your hands and provide privacy.
- Inform the patient that you may reposition the device frequently to
hear the loudest fetal heart sounds.
- Help the patient to the supine position and expose her abdomen, using
a bath blanket to minimize exposure.
- Apply a water-soluble lubricant to her abdomen or to the monitoring
device.
- Apply the device. (See *Assessing fetal heart rate*, page 182.)

Doppler ultrasound stethoscope

- Place the earpieces in your ears or if there are no earpieces, turn on the
device and adjust the volume.
- Press the bell or transducer gently on the abdomen.

ASSESSING FETAL HEART RATE

Fetal heart rate provides important information about fetal well-being. It can be assessed by auscultating the patient's abdomen with a fetoscope or a Doppler ultrasound stethoscope.

FETOSCOPE

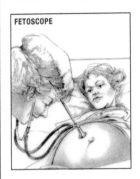

DOPPLER ULTRASOUND STETHOSCOPE

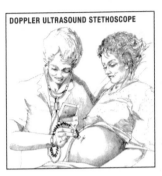

■ Begin to listen at the midline, midway between the umbilicus and symphysis pubis.

Fetoscope

■ Place the earpieces in your ears.
■ Position the fetoscope centrally on your forehead.
■ Gently press the bell about ½" (1 cm) into the patient's abdomen.
■ Remove your hands from the fetoscope to avoid extraneous noise.

Using both methods

■ Move the instrument slightly from side to side to locate the loudest heart sounds.
■ Simultaneously assess the mother's pulse rate for at least 15 seconds.
■ If the maternal pulse rate and FHR are the same, reposition the device slightly and listen again.
■ If you encounter difficulty, try to locate the fetal thorax by using Leopold's maneuvers.

NURSING CONSIDERATIONS

■ Allow the mother and her family to listen to the fetal heart rate if they wish and document their participation.

- After placing the device and locating the fetal heart sounds, monitor maternal and fetal heartbeats for 60 seconds.
- During labor, assess FHR during the relaxation period between contractions to establish a baseline.
- In a low-risk labor, assess FHR every 60 minutes during the latent phase, every 30 minutes during the active phase, and every 15 minutes during the second stage of labor.
- In a high-risk labor, assess FHR every 30 minutes during the latent phase, every 15 minutes during the active phase, and every 5 minutes during the second stage of labor.
- Auscultate FHR during a contraction and for 30 seconds afterward to identify the fetal response to the contraction.
- Always auscultate FHR before administration of medications, ambulation, and artificial rupture of membranes. Also auscultate FHR after rupture of membranes, changes in the characteristics of the contractions, performing vaginal examinations, and administering medications.

ALERT *Notify the physician or nurse-midwife immediately if you observe marked changes in FHR from baseline values, especially during or immediately after a contraction, when signs of fetal distress typically occur. If fetal distress occurs, expect to institute continuous external or internal electronic fetal monitoring.*

- Document FHR and maternal pulse and each auscultation.

Fetal station measurement

DESCRIPTION

- Relationship of the presenting part of the fetus to the mother's ischial spines
- Fetal station of 0 indicative of presenting part at the level of the ischial spines; termed *engagement*
- Measurement in centimeters; labeled as "minus" when the part is above the ischial spines and "plus" when below the level
- Measurements ranging from −1 to −5 cm (minus station) to +1 to +5 cm (plus station) (see *Measuring fetal station*, page 184)
- +4 fetal station indicative of fetal presenting part at the perineum; termed *crowning*

MEASURING FETAL STATION

Fetal station, determined by vaginal examination, is the relationship of the presenting part to the ischial spines. In *engagement*, the presenting part of the fetus is at the level of the mother's ischial spines. In *crowning*, the presenting part of the fetus is at the perineum.

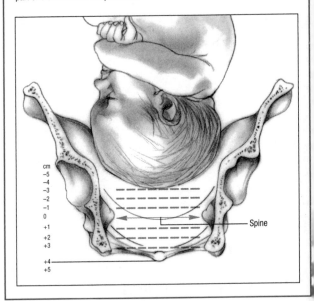

EQUIPMENT

Sterile gloves ◆ sterile water-soluble lubricant or sterile water ◆ mild soap and water or cleaning solution ◆ linen-saver pads

ESSENTIAL STEPS

- Confirm the patient's identity by using two patient identifiers according to facility policy.
- Prepare the patient for a vaginal examination.
- Explain the procedure to the patient and ask her to empty her bladder.
- Identify fetal presenting part and position using Leopold's maneuvers.

- Help the patient into a lithotomy position. Place a linen-saver pad under her buttocks.
- Put on sterile gloves, and lubricate the index and middle fingers of your examining hand with sterile water or sterile water-soluble lubricant. If the membranes are ruptured, use an antiseptic solution.
- Ask the patient to relax by taking several deep breaths and slowly releasing the air.
- Insert lubricated fingers (palmar surface down) into the vagina. Keep your uninserted fingers flexed to avoid the rectum.
- Locate the ischial spines typically palpated as notches at the 4 o'clock and 8 o'clock positions at the pelvic outlet.
- Determine the extent of the fetal presenting part into the pelvis.
- Palpate the presenting part of the fetus and determine the number of centimeters above to below the ischial spines

   ALERT *If the presenting part isn't fully engaged into the pelvis, you won't be able to assess fetal station.*

- Withdraw your fingers gently and wipe away any secretions, lubrication, or examining solution.
- Help the patient clean her perineum, and change the linen-saver pad, as necessary.
- Reposition the patient comfortably.

NURSING CONSIDERATIONS

- Keep in mind that fetal station assessment is commonly done during a vaginal examination in conjunction with assessing cervical dilation and effacement and fetal presentation and position.
- Adhere to standard precautions at all times.
- Don't perform the examination if bleeding is present or if there's evidence of the umbilical cord in the perineal area.
- Document your findings and how the patient tolerated the procedure.

Fundal height measurement

DESCRIPTION

- Reflects the progress of fetal growth and provides a gross estimate of the duration of the pregnancy
- Measurement less than expected for gestational age: intrauterine growth restriction

MEASURING FUNDAL HEIGHT

Typically, between the 20th and 32nd weeks of gestation, the fundal height in centimeters corresponds to the week of gestation. Fundal heights greater than or less than the gestational week may suggest a complication. For example, if the fundal height is significantly greater than what's expected, the patient may have a multiple pregnancy, polyhydramnios or a large-for-gestational-age fetus, or her estimated date of delivery may have been miscalculated. If the measurement is less than what's expected, a small-for-gestational-age fetus, intrauterine growth restriction, or an anomaly may be suspected.

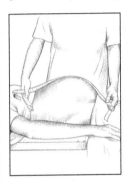 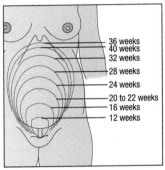

- 36 weeks
- 40 weeks
- 32 weeks
- 28 weeks
- 24 weeks
- 20 to 22 weeks
- 16 weeks
- 12 weeks

- Measurement greater than expected for gestational age: multiple pregnancy, hydramnios
- Locations for palpation/measurement:
  – just over the symphysis pubis at 12 to 14 weeks' gestation
  – at the umbilicus at 20 to 22 weeks' gestation
  – at the xiphoid process at 36 weeks' gestation
- Highest at about 36 weeks' gestation; drops about 4 cm by 40 weeks' gestation, when lightening occurs

EQUIPMENT

Pliable nonstretchable tape measure or pelvimeter ◆ bath blanket

ESSENTIAL STEPS

- Confirm the patient's identity by using two patient identifiers according to facility policy.

- Explain the procedure to the patient and wash your hands.
- Help the patient into a supine position and drape her appropriately with a bath blanket to provide privacy; expose her abdomen.
- Position one end of the tape measure at the notch of the symphysis pubis. (See *Measuring fundal height.*)
- Pull the tape measure up and over the patient's abdomen to the top of the fundus, being careful not to tip the corpus of the fundus back.
- Measure the distance in centimeters.

NURSING CONSIDERATIONS

- During the second and third trimesters, make the measurement more precise by using McDonald's rule to determine the duration of the pregnancy in either lunar months or weeks.
- To calculate the duration in lunar months, multiply the fundal height in centimeters by $2/7$.
- To calculate the duration in weeks, multiply the fundal height in centimeters by $8/7$.
- Plot the measurement on a graph to help identify changes that warrant investigation.

Fundal palpation (postpartum)
DESCRIPTION

- Helps to determine involution: postpartum uterine size, degree of firmness, and rate of descent
- Measured in fingerbreadths above or below the umbilicus
- Typical uterine location: midline
- Typical fundal locations:
  - midway between the umbilicus and symphysis pubis 1 to 2 hours after delivery
  - 1 cm above or at the level of the umbilicus 12 hours after delivery
  - about 3 cm below the umbilicus by the third day after delivery
- Fundal descent: about 1 cm/day until it isn't palpable above the symphysis pubis (about 9 days after delivery)
- Uterine shrinkage: prepregnancy size by about 5 to 6 weeks after delivery (not from a decrease in the number of cells but from a decrease in their size)

PALPATING THE FUNDUS

The illustration below shows how to position your hands to palpate the uterus.

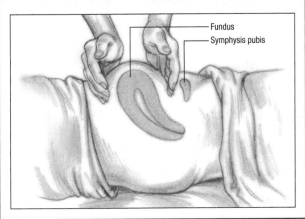

Fundus
Symphysis pubis

EQUIPMENT

Gloves ◆ perineal pad ◆ urinary catheter (optional)

ESSENTIAL STEPS

- Before palpating the uterus, explain the procedure to the patient and provide privacy.
- Confirm the patient's identity by using two patient identifiers according to facility policy.
- Wash your hands and put on gloves.
- Ask the patient to urinate. If she's unable to urinate, anticipate the need to catheterize her.
- Lower the head of the bed until the patient is in a supine position or her head is slightly elevated.
- Expose the abdomen for palpation and the perineum for inspection.

   ALERT Watch for bleeding, clots, and tissue expulsion while massaging the uterus.
- Gently compress the uterus between both hands to evaluate uterine firmness. (See *Palpating the fundus.*)

ALERT *A full-term pregnancy stretches the ligaments supporting the uterus, placing the uterus at risk for inversion during palpation and massage. To guard against this, place one hand against the patient's abdomen at the symphysis pubis level. This steadies the fundus and prevents downward displacement. Then place the other hand at the top of the fundus, cupping it.*

- Note the level of the fundus above or below the umbilicus in centimeters or fingerbreadths.
- If the uterus seems soft and boggy, gently massage the fundus with a circular motion until it becomes firm. Without digging into the abdomen, gently compress and release, always supporting the lower uterine segment with the other hand. Observe the vaginal drainage during massage.
- Massage long enough to produce firmness but not discomfort.

NURSING CONSIDERATIONS

- Check the tone and location of the fundus (the uppermost portion of the uterus) every 15 minutes for the first hour after delivery, every 30 minutes for the next 2 to 3 hours, every hour for the next 4 hours, every 4 hours for the rest of the first postpartum day, and then every 8 hours until the patient is discharged.
- Keep in mind that a firm uterus helps control postpartum hemorrhage by clamping down on uterine blood vessels.
- Assess the patient for bladder distention.

ALERT *Suspect a distended bladder if the uterus isn't firm at the midline; a distended bladder can impede the downward descent of the uterus by pushing it upward and, possibly, to the side.*

- If the fundus feels boggy (soft), massage it gently; if the fundus doesn't respond, a firmer touch should be used.

ALERT *Notify the physician or nurse-midwife immediately if the uterus fails to contract and heavy bleeding occurs. Be prepared to administer oxytocin (Pitocin), ergonovine (Ergotrate), or methylergonovine (Methergine) to maintain uterine firmness as ordered. Be alert for uterine relaxation, which may occur if the uterus relaxes from overstimulation because of massage or medication.*

- For the patient who has had a cesarean delivery, keep in mind that pain at the incision site makes fundal assessment especially uncomfortable. Provide pain medication beforehand as ordered.

Internal electronic fetal monitoring

DESCRIPTION

- Invasive procedure that uses an internal spiral electrode (ISE) attached to the presenting fetal part (usually the scalp) and a fluid-filled intra-uterine pressure catheter (IUPC) inserted into the uterine cavity alongside the fetus
- Detection of fetal heartbeat by spiral electrode with transmission to the monitor, converting the signal to a fetal electrocardiogram (ECG) waveform
- Application of ISE to epidermis of the presenting part to provide a continuous recording of the fetal heart rate (FHR)
- Demonstration of accurate baseline, true baseline variability, and periodic changes (transient and recurrent changes from baseline rates that are associated with uterine contractions)
- Indicated for high-risk pregnancies

   ALERT *Direct electronic fetal monitoring is indicated with rupture of amniotic membranes, cervical dilation of at least 2 cm, and presenting part at least at the −1 station.*

- Risk of maternal complications, including uterine perforation and intrauterine infections
- Risk of fetal complications, including abscess, hematoma, and infection
- Removal of intrauterine pressure catheter usually during the second stage of labor
- Also called *direct monitoring*

EQUIPMENT

Electronic fetal monitor and operating instructions ◆ spiral electrode and drive tube ◆ disposable leg pad or reusable leg pad with Velcro belt ◆ conduction gel ◆ antiseptic solution ◆ hypoallergenic tape ◆ sterile gloves ◆ sterile drapes ◆ intrauterine catheter connection cable and pressure sensitive catheter ◆ graph paper

PERFORMING INTERNAL FETAL MONITORING

The illustration below shows how internal fetal monitoring works.

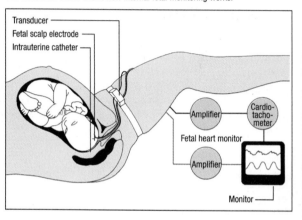

ESSENTIAL STEPS

- Confirm the patient's identity by using two patient identifiers according to facility policy.
- Explain the procedure to the patient.
- Label the printout paper with the patient's identification number or name and birth date, the test date, the paper speed, and the number on the monitor strip.
- Help the patient into the lithotomy position for a vaginal examination.
- Attach the connection cable to the outlet on the monitor marked UA (uterine activity); connect the cable to the intrauterine catheter, and then zero the catheter with a gauge on the distal end of the catheter.
- Cover the patient's perineum with a sterile drape and clean the perineum according to facility policy.
- Assist the health care provider in performing a vaginal examination to insert the intrauterine catheter into the uterine cavity and to attach the fetal scalp electrode to the fetus. (See *Performing internal fetal monitoring*.)

- Secure the catheter and electrode to the leg plate transducer.
- Observe the monitoring strip to verify proper placement and a clear tracing.
- Periodically evaluate the strip to determine the amount of pressure exerted with each contraction. Note all such data on the strip and the patient's medical record.
- To monitor the FHR, apply conduction gel to the leg plate transducer and secure to the patient's inner thigh with Velcro straps or 2" tape; connect the leg plate cable to the electrocardiogram outlet on the monitor.
- Assist with continued examination to identify the fetal presenting part and level of descent. The health care provider will place the spiral electrode in a drive tube and advance it through the vagina to the presenting part; expect mild pressure to be applied and the drive tube to be turned clockwise 360 degrees to secure it.
- Connect the color-coded electrode wires to the corresponding color-coded leg plate posts after the electrode is in place and the drive tube has been removed.
- Turn on the recorder and note the time on the printout paper.
- Help the patient into a comfortable position and evaluate the strip to verify proper placement and a clear FHR tracing.

NURSING CONSIDERATIONS

- Check the baseline FHR, and assess periodic accelerations or decelerations from the baseline. Compare the FHR pattern with the uterine contraction pattern. Note the interval between the onset of deceleration and uterine contractions, the interval between the lowest level of an FHR deceleration and the peak of a uterine contraction, and the range of FHR deceleration.
- Check for FHR variability, which is a measure of fetal oxygen reserve and neurologic integrity and stability.
- Interpret FHR and uterine contractions at regular intervals.
- Adhere to the Guidelines of the Association of Women's Health, Obstetric, and Neonatal Nurses for assessment: high-risk patients need continuous FHR monitoring, whereas low-risk patients should have FHR auscultated every 30 minutes after a contraction during the first stage and every 15 minutes after a contraction during the second stage. First, determine the baseline FHR within 10 beats/minute; then assess the degree of baseline variability. Identify such changes as decel-

erations (early, late, variable, or mixed) and such nonperiodic changes
as a sinusoidal pattern.

⚡ ***ALERT*** *If vaginal delivery isn't imminent (within 30 min-*
utes) and fetal distress patterns are identified, prepare for
an emergency cesarean delivery.

■ Document all activity related to monitoring, maternal vital signs, pushing efforts, use of medications, cervical dilation and effacement, fetal
station, presentation, and position. Also record time of membrane rupture and whether it was spontaneous or artificial.

Leopold's maneuvers
DESCRIPTION

■ Method of determining fetal position, presentation, and attitude
■ Abdominal palpation involving four maneuvers

EQUIPMENT

None

ESSENTIAL STEPS

■ Confirm the patient's identity by using two patient identifiers according to facility policy.
■ Explain the procedure to the patient and ask her to empty her bladder.
■ Wash your hands.
■ Help the patient into a supine position and expose her abdomen while
maintaining her privacy.
■ Perform the first maneuver. (See *Performing Leopold's maneuvers,* page
194.)
  Face the patient and curl your fingers around the fundus. With the fetus in vertex position, the buttocks feel irregularly shaped and firm. With
the fetus in breech position, the head feels hard, round, and movable.
■ Perform the second maneuver.
  Move your hands down the sides of the abdomen, and apply gentle
pressure. If the fetus lies in vertex position, you'll feel a smooth, hard
surface on one side — the fetal back. Opposite, you'll feel lumps and
knobs — the knees, hands, feet, and elbows. If the fetus lies in breech position, you may not feel the back at all.

PERFORMING LEOPOLD'S MANEUVERS

The illustrations below show how the hands are placed on the mother's abdomen for each maneuver.

FIRST MANEUVER

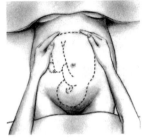

THIRD MANEUVER

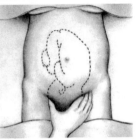

SECOND MANEUVER

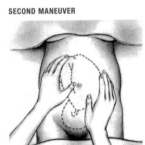

FOURTH MANEUVER

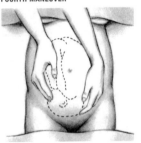

■ Perform the third maneuver.

Spread apart the thumb and fingers of one hand. Place them just above the patient's symphysis pubis. Bring your fingers together. If the fetus lies in vertex position and hasn't descended, you'll feel the head. If the fetus lies in vertex position and has descended, you'll feel a less distinct mass.

■ Perform the fourth maneuver in late pregnancy,

To determine flexion or extension of the fetal head and neck, place your hands on both sides of the lower abdomen. Apply gentle pressure with your fingers as you slide your hands downward, toward the symphysis pubis. If the head presents, one hand's descent will be stopped by the cephalic prominence. The other hand will be unobstructed.

NURSING CONSIDERATIONS

■ Warm your hands before attempting to perform the procedure.
■ Keep in mind the purpose of each maneuver: the first maneuver identifies the occupying fetal part; the second maneuver identifies the fetal back; the third maneuver identifies the fetal presenting part over the inlet; and the fourth maneuver identifies whether or not the head is flexed.
■ Document your findings in the patient's medical record.

Lochia flow assessment
DESCRIPTION

■ Vaginal discharge that occurs after birth; consists of blood, fragments of the decidua, white blood cells (WBCs), mucus, and some bacteria
■ Outermost layer of the uterus that becomes necrotic
■ Categories:
  – *rubra:* red vaginal discharge with fleshy odor and small clots that occurs during the first 3 days after delivery
  – *serosa:* pinkish brown serosanguinous discharge with fleshy odor that occurs during days 4 to 9
  – *alba:* yellow to white vaginal discharge that usually begins about 10 days after delivery and can last from 2 to 6 weeks
■ Commonly assessed in conjunction with fundal assessment

EQUIPMENT

Gloves ◆ perineal pad ◆ linen-saver pad ◆ perineal care supplies, such as peri bottle, soap, water, and washcloth

ESSENTIAL STEPS

■ Confirm the patient's identity by using two patient identifiers according to facility policy.
■ Explain the procedure to the patient.
■ Wash your hands and provide privacy.
■ Help the patient into the lateral Sims' position.
■ Put on gloves and then inspect the perineal pad.

ASSESSING LOCHIA FLOW

Use these guidelines when assessing a patient's lochia.

■ **Character:** Lochia typically is described as lochia rubra, serosa, or alba, depending on the color of the discharge. Lochia should always be present during the first 3 weeks postpartum. The patient who has had a cesarean delivery may have a scant amount of lochia; however, lochia is never absent.

■ **Amount:** Although this varies, the amount can be compared to that of a menstrual flow. Saturating a perineal pad in less than 1 hour is considered excessive; the physician should be notified. Lochia flow increases with activity; for example, when the patient gets out of bed the first several times (due to pooled lochia being released) after delivery or engages in strenuous exercise, such as lifting a heavy object or walking up stairs (due to an actual increase in amount). Expect a patient who is breast-feeding to have a lighter flow of lochia.

■ **Color:** Depending on the postpartum day, lochia typically ranges from red to pinkish brown to creamy white or colorless. A sudden change in the color of lochia — for example, to bright red after having been pink — suggests new bleeding or retained placental fragments.

■ **Odor:** Lochia's odor is similar to that of menstrual flow. Any foul or offensive odor suggests infection.

■ **Consistency:** Lochia should be clot-free. Evidence of large clots indicates poor uterine contraction, which requires intervention.

ALERT *Before removing the perineal pad, make sure that it isn't adhering to any perineal stitches; otherwise, tearing may occur, possibly increasing the risk of bleeding.*

■ Remove the patient's perineal pad and evaluate the character, amount, color, odor, and consistency (presence of clots) of the discharge. (See *Assessing lochia flow.*)

■ Be sure to check under the patient's buttocks to make sure that blood isn't pooling there.

■ Assist the patient with performing perineal care and applying a new perineal pad.

■ Reposition the patient comfortably.

■ Dispose of the used pad according to your facility's policy, remove gloves, and wash hands.

NURSING CONSIDERATIONS

■ Assess lochia along with the fundus every 15 minutes during the first hour after delivery, every 30 minutes for the next 2 to 3 hours, every hour for the next 4 hours, every 4 hours for the rest of the first post-partum day, and then every 8 hours until the patient is discharged.

    ALERT *Watch for continuous seepage of bright red blood, which may indicate a cervical or vaginal laceration; additional evaluation is necessary. Lochia that saturates a sanitary pad within 45 minutes usually indicates an abnormally heavy flow. Weigh perineal pads to estimate the amount of blood loss and always look under the patient's buttocks, where blood may pool.*

- Be alert for an increase in lochia flow on arising; a heavier flow of lochia may occur when the patient first rises from bed because of pooling of the lochia in the vagina.
- Evaluate the amount of clots; numerous large clots require further evaluation because they may interfere with involution.
- Remember that breast-feeding and exertion may increase lochia flow.
- Know that lochia may be scant but should never be absent; this may indicate a postpartum infection.

Neonatal size and weight measurements

DESCRIPTION

- Establishes a baseline for monitoring growth
- Can also be used to detect such disorders as failure to thrive and hydrocephalus
- Include head circumference, chest circumference, head-to-heel length, weight, and abdominal girth

EQUIPMENT

Crib or examination table with a firm surface ◆ scale with tray and scale paper ◆ tape measure ◆ length board ◆ gloves, if neonate hasn't been bathed yet

ESSENTIAL STEPS

- Confirm the patient's identity by using two patient identifiers according to facility policy.
- Explain the procedure to the family if they're present.

OBTAINING ACCURATE SIZE MEASUREMENTS

Accurate measurements are essential to establish a baseline for monitoring normal growth. The illustrations below demonstrate how to obtain accurate head and chest circumferences and head-to-heel length.

MEASURING HEAD CIRCUMFERENCE

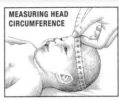

MEASURING CHEST CIRCUMFERENCE

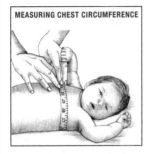

MEASURING HEAD-TO-HEEL LENGTH

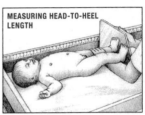

- Wash your hands and put on gloves if the neonate hasn't yet been bathed.
- Position the neonate in a supine position in the crib or on the examination table.
- Remove the neonate's clothing.
- Measure head circumference: Slide the tape measure under the neonate's head at the occiput and draw the tape around snugly, just above the eyebrows. Normal neonatal head circumference is 13″ to 14″ (33 to 35.5 cm). Cranial molding or caput succedaneum from a vaginal delivery may affect this measurement. (See *Obtaining accurate size measurements.*)
- Measure chest circumference: Place tape under the back, wrapping it snugly around the chest at the nipple line, and keeping the back and front of the tape level. Take the measurement after the neonate inspires and before he begins to exhale. Normal neonatal chest circumference is 12″ to 13″ (30.5 to 33 cm).
- Measure head-to-heel length: Fully extend the neonate's legs with the toes pointing up. Measure the distance from the heel to the top of the head. A length board may be used, if available. Normal length is 18″ to 21″ (46 to 53 cm).

- Weight: Remove the diaper and place the neonate in the middle of the scale tray. Keep one hand poised over the neonate at all times. Average weight is 2,500 to 4,000 g (5 lb, 8 oz to 8 lb, 13 oz).
- Measure abdominal girth: Place the tape measure around the abdominal area just about the umbilicus, making sure to keep the tape level.
- Dress and diaper the neonate and return him to his crib or family who can hold and comfort him.

NURSING CONSIDERATIONS

- Always weigh a neonate before a feeding and ensure that the scale is balanced.
- Take the neonate's weight at the same time each day, if possible.
- Throughout measurements, institute measures to minimize heat loss.
- Document your findings and be sure to record whether the neonate had any clothing or equipment on him (such as an I.V.).

Neonatal thermoregulation

DESCRIPTION

- Metabolism of brown fat, which is unique to neonates and has a greater concentration of energy-producing mitochondria in its cells, enhancing its capacity for heat production; effective, but only within a very narrow temperature range
- Provides a neutral thermal environment that helps the neonate maintain a normal core temperature with minimal oxygen consumption and caloric expenditure
- Without careful external thermoregulation: chill can result in hypoxia, acidosis, hypoglycemia, pulmonary vasoconstriction, and death
- Factors making neonates susceptible to hypothermia: relatively large surface-to-weight ratio, reduced metabolism per unit area, and small amounts of insulating fat
- Core temperature: varies, but is approximately 97.7° F (36.5° C); cold stress and its complications preventable with proper interventions

EQUIPMENT

Radiant warmer or incubator (if necessary) (see *Understanding thermoregulators*, page 200) ◆ blankets ◆ washcloths or towels ◆ skin probe ◆ adhesive pad ◆ water-soluble lubricant ◆ thermometer ◆ clothing, including cap

UNDERSTANDING THERMOREGULATORS

Thermoregulators preserve neonatal body warmth in various ways. A radiant warmer maintains the neonate's temperature by radiation. An incubator maintains the neonate's temperature by conduction and convection.

Temperature settings

Radiant warmers and incubators have two operating modes: nonservo and servo. The nurse manually sets the temperature on nonservo equipment; a probe on the neonate's skin controls the temperature settings on servo models.

RADIANT WARMER

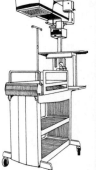

Other features

Most thermoregulators come with alarms. Incubators have the added advantage of providing a stable, enclosed environment, which protects the neonate from evaporative heat loss.

INCUBATOR

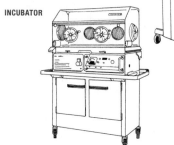

ESSENTIAL STEPS

- While preparing for the neonate's birth, turn on the radiant warmer in the birthing room and set it to the desired temperature. Warm the blankets, washcloths, or towels under a heat source.
- In the birthing room, place the neonate under the radiant warmer, dry him with warm washcloths or towels, and then cover his head with a cap to prevent heat loss.
- Perform required procedures quickly and wrap the neonate in the warmed blankets. If his condition permits, give him to his family to promote bonding.

- Transport the neonate to the nursery in the warmed blankets; use a transport incubator.
- In the nursery, remove the blankets and cap and place the neonate under the radiant warmer.
- Use the adhesive pad to attach the temperature control probe to his skin in the upper-right abdominal quadrant. If the neonate will lie prone, put the skin probe on his back.

  ALERT *Don't cover the device with anything because this could interfere with the servo control.*

- Take the neonate's axillary temperature on admission, every 15 to 30 minutes thereafter until the temperature stabilizes, then every 4 hours to ensure stability.

Incubator use

- Apply a skin probe to a neonate in an incubator as you would for a neonate in a radiant warmer.
- Move the incubator away from cold walls or objects. Perform all required procedures quickly and close portholes in the hood after completion.
- If procedures must be performed outside the incubator, do them under a radiant warmer.
- To leave the facility or to move to a bassinet, a neonate must be weaned from the incubator by slowly reducing the temperature to that of the nursery. Check periodically for hypothermia. When the neonate's temperature stabilizes, dress him, put him in a bassinet, and cover him with a blanket.

NURSING CONSIDERATIONS

- Sponge bathe the neonate under the warmer only after his temperature stabilizes and his glucose level is normal. Leave him under the warmer until his temperature remains stable.

  ALERT *If the temperature doesn't stabilize, place the neonate under a plastic heat shield or in a warmed incubator, according to facility policy. Check for signs of infection, which can cause hypothermia.*

- Use measures to prevent heat loss in the neonate. (See *Preventing heat loss,* page 202.)
- Instruct the family on the importance of and measures for maintaining body temperature.

PREVENTING HEAT LOSS

Follow these steps to prevent heat loss in the neonate.

Conduction
- Preheat the radiant warmer bed and linen.
- Warm stethoscopes and other instruments before use.
- Before weighing the neonate, pad the scale with a paper towel or a preweighed, warmed sheet.

Convection
- Place the neonate's bed out of a direct line with an open window, fan, or air-conditioning vent.

Evaporation
- Dry the neonate immediately after delivery.
- When bathing the neonate, expose only one body part at a time; wash each part thoroughly and then dry it immediately.

Radiation
- Keep the neonate and examining tables away from outside windows and air conditioners.

- Document the name and temperature of the heat source used, the neonate's temperature, and any complications resulting from use of thermoregulatory equipment.

Oxytocin administration

DESCRIPTION

- Used to induce or augment labor (see also "Labor induction and augmentation," page 160.)
- Indications: patients with gestational hypertension, prolonged gestation, maternal diabetes, Rh sensitization, premature or prolonged rupture of membranes, and incomplete or inevitable abortion
- Additional indications: to evaluate for fetal distress after 31 weeks' gestation and to control bleeding and enhance uterine contractions after the placenta is delivered
- Administered I.V. with an infusion pump

   ALERT *Throughout administration, fetal heart rate (FHR) and uterine contractions should be assessed and monitored to ensure that they're occurring in a 20-minute span.*

EQUIPMENT

Administration set for primary I.V. line ◆ infusion pump and tubing ◆ I.V. solution as ordered ◆ external or internal electronic monitoring equipment ◆ oxytocin ◆ label ◆ venipuncture equipment

ESSENTIAL STEPS

- Prepare the oxytocin solution as ordered and label the I.V. container appropriately.
- Confirm the patient's identity by using two patient identifiers according to facility policy.
- Explain the procedure and rationale to the patient.
- Wash your hands and follow standard precautions.
- Insert the tubing of the administration set through the infusion pump, and set the pump to administer the oxytocin according to facility policy.
- Set up the equipment for electronic fetal monitoring.
- Assist the patient to a lateral tilt position and support her hip with a pillow.
- Identify and record FHR and assess uterine contractions occurring in a 20-minute span.
- Start a primary I.V. line if one isn't already in place.
- Piggyback the oxytocin infusion to the primary I.V. line at the Y-injection site closest to the patient
- Begin the oxytocin infusion at the prescribed rate. The typical recommended starting dose is 0.5 to 1.0 mU/minute. The maximum dosage of oxytocin is 20 to 40 mU/minute.
- Because oxytocin begins acting immediately, be prepared to start monitoring uterine contractions.
- Increase oxytocin dosage as ordered.

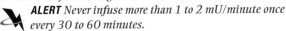 **ALERT** *Never infuse more than 1 to 2 mU/minute once every 30 to 60 minutes.*

NURSING CONSIDERATIONS

- Before each increase, assess contractions, maternal vital signs, and fetal heart rhythm and rate. When using an external fetal monitor, the uterine activity strip or grid should show contractions occurring every 2 to 3 minutes. The contractions should last for about 60 seconds and be

COMPLICATIONS OF OXYTOCIN ADMINISTRATION

Oxytocin can cause uterine hyperstimulation. This, in turn, may progress to tetanic contractions, which last longer than 2 minutes. Signs of hyperstimulation include contractions that are less than 2 minutes apart and last 90 seconds or longer, uterine pressure that doesn't return to baseline between contractions, and intrauterine pressure that rises over 75 mm Hg.

What else to watch for

Other potential complications include fetal distress, abruptio placentae, uterine rupture, and water intoxication. Water intoxication, which can cause maternal seizures or coma, can result because the antidiuretic effect of oxytocin causes decreased urine flow.

Indications for discontinuing drug

Watch for the following signs of oxytocin administration complications. If any indication of any potential complications exists, stop the oxytocin administration, administer oxygen via face mask, and notify the doctor immediately.

Fetal distress
Signs of fetal distress include:
- late decelerations
- bradycardia.

Abruptio placentae
Signs of abruptio placentae include:
- sharp, stabbing uterine pain
- pain over and above the uterine contraction pain
- heavy bleeding
- hard, boardlike uterus.

Also watch for signs of shock, including falling blood pressure, cold and clammy skin, dilation of the nostrils, and rapid, weak pulse.

Uterine rupture
Signs of uterine rupture include:
- sudden, severe pain during a uterine contraction
- tearing sensation
- absent fetal heart sounds.

Also watch for signs of shock, including falling blood pressure, cold and clammy skin, dilation of the nostrils, and rapid, weak pulse.

Water intoxication
Signs and symptoms of water intoxication include:
- headache and vomiting (usually seen first)
- hypertension
- peripheral edema
- shallow or labored breathing
- dyspnea
- tachypnea
- lethargy
- confusion
- change in level of consciousness.

followed by uterine relaxation. When using an internal fetal monitor, look for an optimal baseline value ranging from 5 to 15 mm Hg. The goal is to verify uterine relaxation between contractions.

- Assist with comfort measures, such as repositioning the patient on her other side as needed.
- Continue assessing maternal and fetal responses to the oxytocin.

ALERT *If a problem occurs, such as decelerations of FHR or fetal distress, stop the piggyback infusion immediately and resume the primary line.*

- Review the infusion rate to prevent uterine hyperstimulation. To manage hyperstimulation, discontinue the infusion and administer oxygen. (See *Complications of oxytocin administration.*)
- To reduce uterine irritability, try to increase uterine blood flow. Do this by changing the patient's position and increasing the infusion rate of the primary I.V. line. After hyperstimulation resolves, resume the oxytocin infusion per facility policy.
- Monitor and record intake and output.

ALERT *Output should be at least 30 ml/hour. Oxytocin has an antidiuretic effect at rates of 16 mU/minute and more. Administration of an electrolyte containing I.V. solution may be necessary to maintain electrolyte balance.*

- Document the oxytocin infusion rate, fluid intake and output, FHR, and uterine activity.

Perineal care

DESCRIPTION

- Promotes healing and comfort and prevents infection by cleaning the perineal area
- Performed in conjunction with a perineal assessment and after the patient voids or has a bowel movement
- Two methods: water-jet irrigation system or peri bottle

EQUIPMENT

Gloves ◆ washcloths ◆ clean basin and mild soap ◆ bath blanket ◆ linen-saver pad ◆ perineal pad ◆ peri bottle or irrigation system ◆ bedpan (optional)

ESSENTIAL STEPS

- Confirm the patient's identity by using two patient identifiers according to facility policy.
- Explain the procedure and rationale to the patient.
- Instruct the patient to perform self-perineal care, if she's able.
- Assist the patient to the bathroom or place the patient on a bedpan.
- Wash your hands and put on gloves.
- Remove the patient's perineal pad.

Water-jet system
- Insert the prefilled cartridge containing the antiseptic or medicated solution into the handle, and push the disposable nozzle into the handle until you hear it click into place.
- Help the patient sit on the toilet or bedpan.
- Place the nozzle parallel to the perineum and turn on the unit.
- Rinse the perineum for at least 2 minutes from front to back.
- Turn off the unit, remove the nozzle, and discard the cartridge.
- Dry the nozzle and store as appropriate for later use.

Peri bottle
- Fill the bottle with cleaning solution (usually warm water).
- Help the patient sit on the toilet or bedpan.
- Tell her to pour the solution over her perineal area, or pour the solution over the area for her, ensuring that the solution flows from the front to the back.

Using both methods
- After completion, help the patient off the toilet or remove the bedpan.
- Pat the perineal area dry, and help the patient apply a new perineal pad.
- Dispose of any contaminated supplies according to your facility's policy; clean and dry any reusable equipment.
- Remove gloves and wash your hands.

NURSING CONSIDERATIONS

- During perineal care, inspect the perineal area for signs and symptoms of infection at the episiotomy site, excessive bleeding, or hematoma formation. Report any findings to the physician or nurse-midwife.
- Assess the amount and characteristics of the patient's lochia on her perineal pad. (See "Lochia flow assessment," page 195.)

■ Note whether the patient complains of pain or tenderness. If she does, you may need to apply ice or cold packs to the area for the first 24 hours after birth. This helps reduce perineal edema and prevent hematoma formation, thereby reducing pain and promoting healing.

   ALERT *Cold therapy isn't effective after the first 24 hours. Instead, heat is recommended because it increases circulation to the area. Anticipate the use of a perineal hot pack (dry heat) or a sitz bath (moist heat).*

■ For extensive lacerations, such as third- or fourth-degree lacerations, instruct the patient how to use a sitz bath, which may be ordered to aid perineal healing, provide comfort, and reduce edema.

Phototherapy

DESCRIPTION

■ Exposure of the neonate to high-intensity fluorescent light to break-down bilirubin by oxidation
■ Treatment of choice for hyperbilirubinemia due to hemolytic disease of the neonate (after an initial exchange transfusion)

EQUIPMENT

Phototherapy unit ◆ photometer ◆ eye shields ◆ thermometer ◆ urinometer ◆ surgical face mask or small diaper ◆ thermistor (if phototherapy unit is combined with a temperature-controlled radiant warmer or incubator; optional) ◆ bilimeter

ESSENTIAL STEPS

■ Set up the phototherapy unit about 18″ (45.7 cm) above the neonate's crib, and verify placement of the light bulb shield.
■ If the neonate is in an incubator, place the phototherapy unit at least 3″ (7.6 cm) above the incubator, and turn on the lights.
■ Confirm the neonate's identity by using two patient identifiers according to facility policy.
■ Place a photometer probe in the middle of the crib to measure the energy emitted by the lights. The average range is 6 to 8 uw/cm^2/nanometer.
■ Explain the procedure and rationale to the family.

- Record the neonate's initial bilirubin level and his axillary temperature.
- Place the opaque eye shields over the neonate's closed eyes, and fasten securely.
- Undress the neonate and place a diaper under him. Cover male genitalia with a surgical mask or small diaper to catch urine and prevent possible testicular damage from the heat and light waves.
- Take the neonate's axillary temperature every 2 hours, and provide additional warmth by adjusting the warming unit's thermostat.
- Monitor elimination, and weigh the neonate twice daily. Watch for signs of dehydration (dry skin, poor turgor, depressed fontanels), and check urine specific gravity with a urinometer to gauge hydration status.
- Take the neonate out of the crib, turn off the phototherapy lights, and unmask his eyes at least every 3 to 4 hours (with feedings). Assess his eyes for inflammation or injury.
- Reposition the neonate every 2 hours to expose all body surfaces to the light and to prevent head molding and skin breakdown from pressure.
- Check the bilirubin level at least once every 24 hours — more often if levels rise significantly.
- Turn off the phototherapy unit before drawing venous blood for testing because the lights may degrade bilirubin in the blood.

ALERT *Notify the health care provider if the bilirubin level nears 20 mg/dl if the neonate was born at full term or 15 mg/dl if the neonate was born prematurely.*

NURSING CONSIDERATIONS

- Clean the neonate's eyes periodically to remove drainage.
- Offer the neonate extra water to promote bilirubin excretion.
- Inform the family that the neonate's stool contains some bile and may be green in color.
- Monitor intake and output closely and obtain daily weights to assess fluid balance.
- Encourage the family to hold and cuddle the neonate when out of the bilirubin lights.

RhoGAM administration

DESCRIPTION

- Concentrated solution of immune globulin containing $Rh_o(D)$ antibodies (RhoGAM)
- I.M. injection: keeps Rh-negative mother from producing active antibody responses and forming anti-$Rh_o(D)$ to Rh-positive fetal blood cells and endangering future Rh-positive neonates
- Indicated for Rh-negative mother after abortion, ectopic pregnancy, delivery of a neonate having $Rh_o(D)$-positive or D^u-positive blood and Coombs' negative cord blood, accidental transfusion of Rh-positive blood, amniocentesis, abruptio placentae, or abdominal trauma
- Given within 72 hours to prevent future maternal sensitization
- Also is administered at about 28 weeks' gestation to protect the fetus of the Rh-negative mother

EQUIPMENT

RhoGAM vial ◆ appropriate size of needle and syringe ◆ alcohol or other antiseptic wipe ◆ gloves

ESSENTIAL STEPS

- Confirm the patient's identity by using two patient identifiers according to facility policy.
- Prepare the RhoGAM in the syringe according to the manufacturer's instructions.
- Explain the procedure and rationale for the medication to the patient.
- Wash your hands and provide for privacy.
- Confirm the patient's identity.
- Assist the patient to a comfortable position that will allow access to the gluteal site.
- Cleanse the site with the antiseptic pad and allow the site to air-dry.
- Keep the antiseptic pad nearby for later use.
- Stretch the skin at the site taut with your nondominant hand.
- Remove the needle cover from the needle, and hold the needle and attached syringe at a 90-degree angle.
- Quickly insert the needle into the site and aspirate for blood. If no blood appears, slowly inject the RhoGAM.

- Gently but quickly remove the needle at a 90-degree angle and cover the injection site with the antiseptic pad, applying pressure to the site.
- Dispose of equipment according to your facility's policy.
- Check the vial's identification numbers with another nurse, and sign the triplicate form that comes with the RhoGAM.
- Attach the top copy to the patient's medical record.
- Send the remaining two copies, along with the empty RhoGAM vial, to the laboratory or blood bank.

NURSING CONSIDERATIONS

- Give the patient a card indicating her Rh-negative status and instruct her to carry it with her or keep it in a convenient location.
- Inspect the injection site for active bleeding or bruising.
- Provide comfort measures if the patient complains of pain at the injection site.

Uterine contraction palpation
DESCRIPTION

- Provides information about the frequency, duration, and intensity of contractions and the relaxation time between them
- Character of contractions dependent on stage of labor and body's response to labor-inducing drugs, if administered
- Increased frequency, intensity, and duration of contractions as labor advances

EQUIPMENT

Watch with second hand ◆ bath blanket or sheet for draping

ESSENTIAL STEPS

- Review the patient's history to determine the onset, frequency, duration, and intensity of the contractions, noting where contractions feel strongest or exert the most pressure.
- Wash your hands and provide privacy.
- Confirm the patient's identity by using two patient identifiers according to facility policy.

UNDERSTANDING
UTERINE CONTRACTIONS

As shown below, uterine contractions occur in three phases: increment (building up), acme (peak), and decrement (letting down). Between contractions is a period of relaxation. The two most important features of contractions are duration and frequency. Duration is the elapsed time from the start to the end of one contraction. Frequency refers to the elapsed time from the start of one contraction to the start of the next contraction.

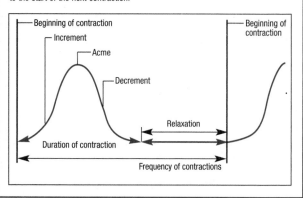

- Explain the procedure to the patient.
- Assist the patient into a comfortable side-lying position.
- Drape the patient with a sheet.
- Place the palmar surface of your fingers on the uterine fundus, and palpate lightly to assess contractions. Each contraction has three phases: increment (rising), acme (peak), and decrement (letting down or ebbing). (See *Understanding uterine contractions.*)
- To assess frequency, time the interval between the beginning of one contraction and the beginning of the next.
- To assess duration, time the period from when the uterus begins tightening until it begins relaxing.
- To assess intensity, press your fingertips into the uterine fundus when the uterus tightens. During mild contractions, the fundus indents easily; during moderate contractions, the fundus indents less easily; during strong contractions, the fundus resists indenting.

- Determine how the patient copes with discomfort by assessing her breathing and relaxation techniques.
- After the contraction subsides, assist the patient to a comfortable position.
- Wash your hands.

NURSING CONSIDERATIONS

- Assess contractions in low-risk patients every 30 minutes in the latent phase, every 15 to 30 minutes in the active phase, and every 15 minutes in the transition phase. Assess high-risk patients more frequently, such as every 30 minutes during the latent phase, every 15 minutes during the active phase, and every 5 minutes in the second stage.
- Provide comfort measures as indicated before, during, and after the contractions.

   ALERT *If any contraction lasts longer than 90 seconds and isn't followed by uterine muscle relaxation, or if the relaxation period is less than 1 minute between contractions, notify the physician or nurse-midwife immediately. This might indicate uterine hyperstimulation or tetanic contractions, which can interrupt uteroplacental blood flow, possibly leading to fetal hypoxia and fetal distress. Position the patient on her left side to improve uteroplacental perfusion, and administer oxygen via face mask to increase fetal oxygenation.*
- Document the frequency, duration, and intensity of the contractions and the relaxation time between contractions. Also record the patient's response to the contractions and measures used to promote comfort.

Vitamin K administration
DESCRIPTION

- Administered prophylactically to all neonates to prevent a transient deficiency of coagulation factors II, VII, IX, and X
- Neonate's GI system at birth: sterile and lacking the necessary flora to manufacture vitamin K, predisposing the neonate to a deficiency of vitamin K, thus placing him at risk for bleeding
- Typical dosage: single dose of 0.5 mg to 1 mg (0.25 ml to 0.5 ml) given via I.M. route in the birthing room or within 1 to 2 hours following birth

SELECTING THE APPROPRIATE I.M. INJECTION SITE

The illustration shown at right highlights the vastus lateralis muscle, the preferred I.M. injection site for vitamin K administration.

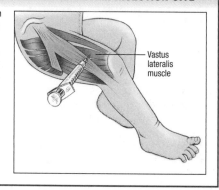

Vastus lateralis muscle

■ Additional dose: may be ordered 6 to 8 hours after birth if the mother received anticoagulant therapy during pregnancy

EQUIPMENT

Prescribed dose of vitamin K ◆ appropriate size syringe with a 23G to 25G, ⅝" safety needle ◆ alcohol or other antiseptic pad ◆ dry gauze pad ◆ gloves

ESSENTIAL STEPS

■ Confirm the neonate's identity by using two patient identifiers according to facility policy.
■ Wash hands and prepare the medication in the syringe according to your facility's policy.
■ Explain the procedure and rationale to the family, if present.
■ Confirm the neonate's identity and place him on a firm, flat surface.
■ Locate the vastus lateralis muscle and select an appropriate site for injection. (See *Selecting the appropriate I.M. injection site.*)

ALERT *Be sure to select a site on the lateral aspect of the neonate's thigh rather than the medial aspect, which can cause the neonate more pain.*

■ Put on clean gloves.

- Clean the intended site with an alcohol or other antiseptic pad and allow the skin to dry.
- Using your nondominant hand, stabilize the leg and grasp the portion of the upper thigh.
- With your dominant hand, quickly insert the needle at a 90-degree angle using a darting action.
- Stabilize the syringe with your nondominant hand and aspirate for blood with your dominant hand.
- If no blood appears, slowly inject the medication.

   ALERT If blood appears in the syringe, don't inject the medication. Withdraw the needle and discard the needle and syringe according to your facility's policy. Prepare a new syringe with medication.

- Withdraw the needle and gently massage the site with a dry gauze pad to increase absorption.
- Remove gloves and discard the used equipment according to your facility's policy.
- Wash your hands.

NURSING CONSIDERATIONS

- Provide comfort to the neonate and his family after injection.
- Monitor the injection site for bleeding, edema, and inflammation.

   ALERT Assess the neonate for bleeding, which may occur on the second or third day. Note bruising or ecchymoses. Inspect umbilical cord area, circumcision, nose, mouth, and GI tract. Monitor prothrombin time and partial thromboplastin time.

- If the vastus lateralis site can't be used, use the rectus femoris site as an alternative. Use this site with caution because it's close to the femoral artery and sciatic nerve.
- If the neonate is to be circumcised, ensure that he has already received vitamin K.
- Document medication administration, including the site of administration, the patient's tolerance to the procedure, and the condition of the injection site.

Part four

Diagnostic tests

Amniotic fluid analysis

PURPOSE

- To detect fetal abnormalities, particularly chromosomal and neural tube defects
- To detect hemolytic disease of the neonate
- To diagnose metabolic disorders, amino acid disorders, and muco-polysaccharidosis
- To determine fetal age and maturity
- To assess fetal health by detecting the presence of meconium or blood or measuring amniotic levels of estriol and fetal thyroid hormone
- To identify fetal gender when one or both parents are carriers of a sex-linked disorder

PATIENT PREPARATION

- Explain the procedure and answer the patient's questions.
- Inform the patient that she need not restrict food and fluids.
- Explain to the patient that she'll feel a stinging sensation when the local anesthetic is injected.
- Ask the patient to void just before the test to minimize the risk of puncturing the bladder.

PROCEDURE

- After determining fetal and placental position, a pool of amniotic fluid is located, usually through palpation and ultrasonic visualization.
- The skin is prepared with antiseptic and alcohol, and 1 ml of 1% lidocaine is injected with a 25G needle, first intradermally and then subcutaneously.
- A 20G spinal needle with a stylet is inserted into the amniotic cavity and the stylet is withdrawn.
- A 20-ml syringe is attached to the needle, after which the fluid is aspirated and placed in an amber or foil-covered test tube.
- The needle is withdrawn and an adhesive bandage placed over the needle insertion site.
- The fetal heart rate (FHR), maternal vital signs, and uterine activity are monitored every 15 minutes for at least 30 minutes.

AMNIOTIC FLUID ANALYSIS FINDINGS

Amniotic fluid analysis can provide information about the condition of the mother, fetus, and placenta. This table shows normal findings and abnormal findings and their implications.

Test component	Normal findings	Fetal implications of abnormal findings
Color	Clear, with white flecks of vernix caseosa in a mature fetus	Blood of maternal origin is usually harmless. "Port wine" fluid may indicate abruptio placentae. Fetal blood may indicate damage to the fetal, placental, or umbilical cord vessels.
Bilirubin	Absent at term	High levels indicate hemolytic disease of the newborn.
Meconium	Absent	Presence indicates fetal hypotension or distress.
Creatinine	More than 2 mg/dl (SI, 177 μmol/L in a mature fetus)	Decrease may indicate fetus less than 37 weeks.
Lecithin-sphingomyelin ratio	More than 2	Less than 2 indicates pulmonary immaturity.
Phosphatidyl glycerol	Present	Absence indicates pulmonary immaturity.
Glucose	Less than 45 mg/dl (SI, 2.3 mmol/L)	Excessive increases at term or near term indicate hypertrophied fetal pancreas.
Alpha-fetoprotein	Variable, depending on gestational age and laboratory technique	Inappropriate increases indicate neural tube defects, such as spina bifida or anencephaly, impending fetal death, congenital nephrosis, or contamination of fetal blood.
Bacteria	Absent	Presence indicates chorioamnionitis.
Chromosome	Normal karyotype	Abnormal karyotype indicates fetal chromosome disorders.
Acetylecholinesterase	Absent	Presence may indicate neural tube defects, exomphalos, or other serious malformations.

POSTPROCEDURE CARE

- Continue to monitor FHR, maternal vital signs, and uterine activity as indicated.
- Assess for possible complications, such as spontaneous abortion, fetal or placental trauma, bleeding, premature labor, infection, and Rh sensitization from fetal bleeding into maternal circulation.
- If the patient is Rh negative, administer RhoD immune globulin (RhoGAM), as ordered, to prevent isoimmunization.
- Before the patient is discharged, instruct her to immediately report abdominal pain or cramping, uterine contractions, chills, fever, vaginal bleeding or leakage of serous vaginal fluid, or fetal hyperactivity or unusual fetal lethargy.
- Encourage the patient to engage in only light activity for 24 hours after amniocentesis to prevent uterine irritability.

NORMAL RESULTS

Clear fluid but may contain white flecks of vernix caseosa when the fetus is near term

ABNORMAL RESULTS

See *Amniotic fluid analysis findings,* page 217.

Biophysical profile

PURPOSE

- To assess fetal well-being in the later stages of pregnancy
- To aid in detecting central nervous system depression in the fetus

PATIENT PREPARATION

- Explain the procedure and its purpose to the patient.
- Inform her that she'll be positioned on her back and that conductive gel will be applied to her lower abdomen.
- Warn the patient that the gel may feel cold.
- Instruct her to drink fluids and avoid urination before the test to ensure a full bladder.
- Reassure the patient that the test won't harm the fetus.

VARIABLES ASSESSED IN A BIOPHYSICAL PROFILE

- Fetal breathing movements
- Fetal body movements
- Fetal muscle tone
- Amniotic fluid volume
- Fetal heart rate reactivity

PROCEDURE

- Position the patient on the examination table in the supine position.
- Coat the lower abdomen with a water-soluble conductive gel.
- The transducer crystal is guided over the area, and images are observed on the scope and photographed.
- The fetus and surrounding structures are visualized.
- Four to six variables are assessed. (See *Variables assessed in a biophysical profile.*)
- Each variable can score a maximum of 2 points.
- The total score is then calculated.
- A nonstress test or contraction stress test may be done simultaneously.

POSTPROCEDURE CARE

- Allow the patient to empty her bladder immediately after the test.
- Remove conductive gel from the patient's abdomen.

NORMAL RESULTS

- Score of 8 to 10: healthy fetus

ABNORMAL RESULTS

- Score of 6: suspicious
- Score of 4: fetus in jeopardy

Chorionic villi sampling

PURPOSE

- To analyze for fetal chromosomal and biochemical abnormalities, such as Tay-Sachs disease, sickle cell disease, anemia, cystic fibrosis, and Down syndrome

CHORIONIC VILLI SAMPLING

Chorionic villi sampling is a prenatal test for quick detection of fetal chromosomal and biochemical disorders that's performed during the first trimester of pregnancy.

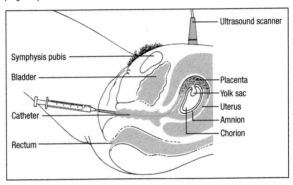

PATIENT PREPARATION

- Explain to the patient that samples are obtained routinely at about 10 to 12 weeks' gestation.
- Tell her that the test involves a vaginal examination and ultrasound.

PROCEDURE

- Assist the patient into the lithotomy position.
- The physician checks placement of the patient's uterus bimanually and then inserts a Graves' speculum and swabs the cervix with an antiseptic solution.
- If necessary, a tenaculum is used to straighten an acutely flexed uterus, permitting cannula insertion.
- Guided by ultrasound and possibly endoscopy, the catheter is inserted transvaginally through the cannula to the villi.
- Suction is applied to the catheter to remove about 30 mg of tissue from the villi.
- A specimen is withdrawn and placed in a Petri dish. It's examined with a dissecting microscope. Part of the specimen is then cultured for further testing. (See *Chorionic villi sampling.*)

POSTPROCEDURE CARE

■ Monitor the patient closely for adverse effects.
■ Be alert for such possible complications as spontaneous abortion, cramps, infection, and bleeding.
■ Instruct the patient to report any cramping, vaginal bleeding or discharge, fever, or lower abdominal pain immediately.
■ If the patient is Rh negative, give RhoGAM as ordered.

NORMAL RESULTS

■ No abnormalities

ABNORMAL RESULTS

■ May indicate more than 200 disorders

Fern test

PURPOSE

■ To confirm amniotic fluid presence and rupture of membranes
■ To differentiate amniotic fluid from urine

PATIENT PREPARATION

■ Confirm the patient's identity by using two patient identifiers according to facility policy.
■ Explain the testing to the patient.
■ Tell her that a sterile vaginal examination will be done to obtain the fluid sample.

PROCEDURE

■ Place the patient in the lithotomy position.
■ Assist with or perform a sterile vaginal examination.
■ Use a sterile, cotton-tipped swab or pipette to obtain fluid from the vagina, and then touch the swab or pipette to the slide.
■ Allow the slide to dry.
■ Observe the slide for evidence of a "ferning" or palmlike leaf pattern under a microscope.

POSTPROCEDURE CARE

- Assist the patient to a comfortable position.
- Assist with measures to support labor progression or halt preterm labor.

NORMAL RESULTS

- Fluid that shows ferning pattern under microscopy

ABNORMAL RESULTS

- Fluid that doesn't show ferning: may be urine rather than amniotic fluid

Human chorionic gonadotropin, serum

PURPOSE

- To detect early pregnancy
- To determine adequacy of hormonal production in high-risk pregnancies (for example, habitual abortion)
- To aid in the diagnosis of trophoblastic tumors, such as hydatidiform mole and choriocarcinoma, and tumors that ectopically secrete human chorionic gonadotropin (hCG)
- To monitor treatment for induction of ovulation and conception

PATIENT PREPARATION

- Confirm the patient's identity by using two patient identifiers according to facility policy.
- Explain to the patient that this test determines whether she's pregnant.
- Inform her that she need not restrict food and fluids.
- Tell the patient that the test requires a blood sample. Explain who will perform the venipuncture and when.
- Explain to the patient that she may experience slight discomfort from the tourniquet and the needle puncture.

PROCEDURE

- Perform a venipuncture and collect the sample according to facility protocol.

- Handle the sample gently to prevent hemolysis.
- Send the sample to the laboratory immediately.

POSTPROCEDURE CARE

- Apply direct pressure to the venipuncture site until bleeding stops.
- Assess for hematoma at the venipuncture site

NORMAL RESULTS

- Less than 4 IU/L
- During pregnancy: hCG levels widely varying, depending partly on the number of days after the last normal menstrual period

ABNORMAL RESULTS

- Positive test in a nonpregnant patient: may indicate ectopic pregnancy, miscarriage, hydatidiform mole, or ovarian cancer

Human chorionic gonadotropin, urine

PURPOSE

- To detect and confirm pregnancy
- To aid in the diagnosis of hydatidiform mole or human chorionic gonadotropin (hCG)–secreting tumors, threatened abortion, or fetal death

PATIENT PREPARATION

- If appropriate, explain to the patient that the urine hCG test determines whether she's pregnant or determines the status of her pregnancy.
- Tell the patient that she need not restrict food but should restrict fluids for 8 hours before the test.
- Inform the patient that the test requires a first-voided morning specimen or urine collection over a 24-hour period, depending on whether the test is qualitative or quantitative.
- Notify the laboratory and physician of drugs the patient is taking that may affect test results; it may be necessary to restrict them.

PROCEDURE

- For verification of pregnancy (qualitative analysis), collect a first-voided morning specimen. If this isn't possible, collect a random specimen.
- For quantitative analysis of hCG, collect the patient's urine over a 24-hour period in the appropriate container, discarding the first specimen and retaining the last.
- Specify the date of the patient's last menstrual period on the laboratory request.
- Refrigerate the 24-hour specimen or keep it on ice during the collection period.
- Make sure the test occurs at least 5 days after a missed period to avoid a false-negative result.

POSTPROCEDURE CARE

- Instruct the patient that she may resume her usual diet and medications.

NORMAL RESULTS

- Qualitative immunoassay analysis: positive results indicate pregnancy
- Quantitative analysis: urine hCG levels in the first trimester of a normal pregnancy up to 500,000 IU/24 hours; in the second trimester, from 10,000 to 25,000 IU/24 hours; in the third trimester, from 5,000 to 15,000 IU/24 hours

ABNORMAL RESULTS

- Abnormal hCG levels: may indicate ectopic pregnancy or miscarriage

Maternal serum alpha-fetoprotein
PURPOSE

- To screen those patients needing amniocentesis or high-resolution ultrasonography during pregnancy

PATIENT PREPARATION

- Explain that this test helps in monitoring fetal development, screens for a need for further testing, helps detect possible congenital defects in the fetus, and monitors the mother's response to therapy by measuring a specific blood protein, as appropriate.

- Inform the patient that she need not restrict food, fluids, or medications.
- Tell the patient that the test requires a blood sample.
- Explain who will perform the venipuncture and when.
- Explain to the patient that she may experience slight discomfort from the tourniquet and the needle puncture.

PROCEDURE

- Confirm the patient's identity by using two patient identifiers according to facility policy.
- Perform a venipuncture and collect the sample according to facility protocol.
- Record the patient's age, race, weight, and week of gestation on the laboratory request.

   ALERT Be sure to determine the specific gestational age in weeks to ensure that the test results are accurate.
- Handle the sample gently to prevent hemolysis.

POSTPROCEDURE CARE

- Apply direct pressure to the venipuncture site until bleeding stops.
- Monitor for signs of hematoma at the venipuncture site.
- Arrange for follow-up ultrasound and amniocentesis as necessary, if results are abnormal.

NORMAL RESULTS

- 25 ng/ml (SI, 25 mcg/L)
- At 15 to 18 weeks' gestation: 10 to 150 ng/ml (SI, 10 to 150 mcg/L)

ABNORMAL RESULTS

   ALERT Alpha-fetoprotein levels rise sharply in 90% of fetuses with anencephaly and in 50% of those with spina bifida. High maternal serum alpha-fetoprotein (MSAFP) levels may indicate intrauterine death or such anomalies as duodenal atresia, omphalocele, tetralogy of Fallot, or Turner's syndrome. Decreased MSAFP levels are associated with Down syndrome.

Nonstress test

PURPOSE

- To screen for suspected fetal distress or placental insufficiency associated with the following maternal conditions: diabetes mellitus, hyperthyroidism, chronic or gestational hypertension, collagen disease, heart disease, chronic renal disease, intrauterine growth restriction, sickle cell disease, Rh sensitization, suspected postmaturity (when the patient is suspected of being past her due date), history of miscarriage or stillbirth, and abnormal estriol excretion

PATIENT PREPARATION

- Explain the purpose and procedure involved with the testing.
- Instruct the patient in how she'll be participating in the test.
- Inform the patient that the test usually is performed over 20 to 40 minutes.

PROCEDURE

- Confirm the patient's identity by using two patient identifiers according to facility policy.
- Obtain baseline vital signs and fetal heart rate (FHR).
- Place the patient in a semi-Fowler or lateral-tilt position with a pillow under one hip.

   ALERT *Avoid placing the patient in the supine position because pressure on the maternal great vessels from the gravid uterus may cause maternal hypotension and reduced uterine perfusion.*

- Apply conductive gel to the abdomen and place transducers on the patient's abdomen to transmit and record FHR and fetal movement.
- Instruct the patient to depress the monitor's mark or test button when she feels the fetus move.
- If no spontaneous fetal movement occurs within 20 minutes, apply gentle pressure to the patient's abdomen or shake it to stimulate fetal movement.
- If gentle pressure is ineffective, use an artificial larynx (vibroacoustic stimulator) to the mother's abdomen to provide a stimulus for 1 to 2 seconds; repeat stimulation for a maximum of three times for up to 3 seconds.

INTERPRETING NST RESULTS

This chart lists the possible interpretations of results from a nonstress test (NST). Appropriate actions are also included.

Result	Interpretation	Action
Reactive	Two or more fetal heart rate (FHR) accelerations of 15 beats/minute lasting 15 seconds or more within 20 minutes; related to fetal movement	Repeat NST biweekly or weekly, depending on rationale for testing.
Nonreactive	Tracing without FHR accelerations or with accelerations of fewer than 15 beats/minute lasting less than 15 seconds throughout fetal movement	Repeat in 24 hours or perform a biophysical profile immediately.
Unsatisfactory	Quality of FHR recording inadequate for interpretation	Repeat in 24 hours or perform a biophysical profile immediately.

POSTPROCEDURE CARE

- Continue to monitor maternal vital signs and fetal heart periodically for changes.
- Inform the patient about the need for any additional follow-up testing.

NORMAL RESULTS

- A reactive nonstress test (NST) that demonstrates an intact fetal autonomic nervous system is controlling FHR: indicated by two FHR accelerations that exceed baseline by at least 15 beats/minute, that last longer than 15 seconds, and that occur within a 20-minute period

  ALERT *If reactive results aren't obtained, the fetus should be monitored for an additional 40 minutes. If reactive NST results still aren't obtained, an oxytocin challenge test (contraction stress test) may be performed to more definitively assess fetal status.*

ABNORMAL RESULTS

See *Interpreting NST results.*

Oxytocin challenge test

PURPOSE

- To evaluate the respiratory functioning of the placenta, providing an indication of how the fetus will tolerate the stress of labor
- To provide further information when a nonstress test is nonreactive

PATIENT PREPARATION

- Explain the purpose and procedure involved with the testing
- Instruct the patient that her contractions and the status of the fetus will be monitored electronically.
- Assess the patient for possible contraindications, such as unexplained third trimester bleeding, preterm labor, placenta previa, and a classic cesarean delivery incision.
- Tell the patient that an I.V. line will be started to administer the oxytocin.
- Assess baseline maternal vital signs and fetal heart rate (FHR).

PROCEDURE

- Confirm the patient's identity by using two patient identifiers according to facility policy.
- Place the patient in a semi-Fowler position or lateral tilt position with a pillow beneath one hip.

ALERT *Avoid placing the patient in the supine position because pressure on the maternal great vessels from the gravid uterus may cause maternal hypotension and reduced uterine perfusion.*

- Start an I.V. infusion with normal saline solution.
- Place a tocotransducer and an ultrasound transducer on the patient's abdomen for 20 minutes to record baseline vital signs and measurements of uterine contractions, fetal movements, and FHR.
- Begin administration of oxytocin as ordered.
- Continue to monitor uterine contractions and FHR and pattern.

ALERT *Be alert for possible uterine hyperstimulation, which could lead to fetal hypoxia. If hyperstimulation occurs, notify the physician immediately and stop the oxytocin.*

- After three contractions are recorded, stop the oxytocin.

INTERPRETING OCT RESULTS

This chart lists the possible interpretations of results from an oxytocin challenge test (OCT), commonly called a stress test. Appropriate actions are also included.

Result	Interpretation	Action
Negative	No late decelerations; three contractions every 10 minutes; fetus would probably survive labor if it occurred within 1 week	No further action needed now.
Positive	Persistent and consistent late decelerations with more than half of contractions	Induce labor; fetus is at risk for perinatal morbidity and mortality.
Suspicious	Late decelerations with less than half of contractions after an adequate contraction pattern has been established	Repeat test in 24 hours.
Hyperstimulation	Late decelerations with excessive uterine activity (occurring more often than every 2 minutes or lasting longer than 90 seconds)	Repeat test in 24 hours.
Unsatisfactory	Poor monitor tracing or uterine contraction pattern	Repeat test in 24 hours.

POSTPROCEDURE CARE

■ Continue to monitor maternal and fetal status for 30 minutes after the oxytocin is stopped or until the contraction rate returns to baseline
■ Offer comfort measures for the patient; reposition the patient as necessary.
■ Continuously assess the patient for signs and symptoms indicating the onset of labor; use of oxytocin may precipitate labor.

NORMAL RESULTS

■ FHR within the normal range of 120 to 160 beats/minute during at least three contractions lasting 40 seconds each, within a 10-minute period without any late decelerations; indicates that the fetus can tolerate the stress of labor

- No late decelerations during each of the three contractions
- Normal or negative oxytocin challenge test: a reassuring finding that there's sufficient placental reserve to supply the fetus during labor contractions

ALERT *Late FHR decelerations during two or more contractions or late decelerations that are inconsistent indicate the risk of fetal hypoxia.*

ABNORMAL RESULTS

See *Interpreting OCT results*, page 229.

Pelvic ultrasound

PURPOSE

- To evaluate fetal viability, position, gestational age, and growth rate
- To detect multiple pregnancy
- To confirm fetal abnormalities (such as molar pregnancy and abnormalities of the arms and legs, spine, heart, head, kidneys, and abdomen)
- To confirm maternal abnormalities (such as posterior placenta and placenta previa)
- To guide amniocentesis by determining placental location and fetal position

PATIENT PREPARATION

- Make sure the patient has signed an appropriate consent form.
- Note and report all allergies.
- Instruct the patient to drink fluids and avoid urination before the test because pelvic ultrasonography requires a full bladder as a landmark to define pelvic organs.
- Explain that the test won't harm the fetus.

PROCEDURE

- With the patient in a supine position, coat the lower abdomen with mineral oil or water-soluble jelly to increase sound wave conduction.
- The transducer crystal is guided over the area, images are observed on the oscilloscope screen, and good images are photographed.

POSTPROCEDURE CARE

- Allow the patient to empty her bladder immediately after the test.
- Remove ultrasound gel from the patient's skin.

NORMAL RESULTS

- During pregnancy: gestational sac and fetus are of normal size for date; placenta located in the fundus of the uterus

ABNORMAL RESULTS

- May indicate fetal abnormalities, such as structural defects (spina bifida), congenital heart defects, or cleft lip and cleft palate

Percutaneous umbilical blood sampling

PURPOSE

- To obtain fetal blood samples for fetal karyotyping
- To aid in identifying hemophilia, hemoglobinopathies, fetal infections, chromosomal abnormalities, fetal distress, and fetal drug levels
- To provide access to fetal circulation for transfusion in utero
- To assess acid-base balance of a fetus with intrauterine growth restriction
- Referred to as *PUBS*

PATIENT PREPARATION

- Make sure the patient has signed an appropriate consent form.
- Explain the purpose, benefits, and risks of the test.
- Ensure that the patient is past her 16th week of gestation.
- Tell the patient that a needle will be inserted into her abdomen.
- Inform her that an ultrasound will be done to help guide the insertion of the needle.
- Assist the patient with measures to promote relaxation.

PROCEDURE

- Assist the patient to the supine position.
- A local anesthetic may be applied to the patient's abdominal wall.

- Apply conductive gel to her abdomen.
- An ultrasound transducer (placed in a sterile glove) scans the abdomen for landmarks.
- A fine needle is inserted through the patient's abdomen and uterine wall into the fetal umbilical vein of the umbilical cord 1 to 2 cm from the cord's insertion site at the placenta.
- A sample of fetal blood is withdrawn into a syringe containing an anti-coagulant and sent to the laboratory for analysis.

POSTPROCEDURE CARE

- Monitor the patient's vital signs frequently, at least every 15 minutes for the first 30 to 60 minutes.
- Assess uterine activity frequently; preterm labor is possible.
- Assess fetal heart rate (FHR) and activity via a nonstress test or external fetal monitoring; report any signs of fetal distress, including fetal bradycardia and nonreassuring FHR patterns.
- Obtain an ultrasound approximately 1 hour after completion of the test to evaluate for possible bleeding at the needle insertion site.

▶ **COLLABORATION** *If the test results indicate an abnormality, prepare the patient and her family for consultations with specialists, such as in genetics or hematology. Provide emotional support and arrange for social service assistance as indicated.*

- If the patient is Rh negative, administer RhoGAM as ordered.
- Encourage the patient to monitor her temperature to determine possible infection.

NORMAL RESULTS

- No abnormalities noted

ABNORMAL RESULTS

- May indicate Rh disease in the fetus, fetal chromosomal defect, or a fetal platelet disorder

Part five

Clinical tools

Cultural childbearing practices

A patient's cultural beliefs can affect her attitudes toward illness and traditional medicine. By trying to accommodate her beliefs and practices in your care plan, you can increase the patient's willingness to learn and comply with treatment regimens. Because cultural beliefs may vary within particular groups, individual practices may differ from those described here.

AFRICAN AMERICANS

- View pregnancy as a state of well-being
- May delay prenatal care
- Believe that taking pictures during pregnancy may cause stillbirth
- Believe that reaching up during pregnancy may cause the umbilical cord to strangle the baby
- May use self-treatment for discomfort
- May cry out during labor or may be stoic
- May receive emotional support during birth from mother or another woman
- May view vaginal bleeding during postpartum period as sickness
- May prohibit tub baths and shampooing hair in the postpartum period
- May view breast-feeding as embarrassing and therefore bottle-feed
- Consider infant who eats well "good"
- May introduce solid food early
- May oil the baby's skin
- May place a bellyband on the neonate to prevent umbilical hernia

ARAB-AMERICANS

- May not seek prenatal care
- Seek medical assistance when medical resources at home fail
- Fast during pregnancy to produce a son
- May labor in silence to be in control
- Limit male involvement during childbirth

ASIAN-AMERICANS

- View pregnancy as a natural process
- Believe mother has "happiness in her body"
- Omit milk from diet because it causes stomach distress
- Believe inactivity and sleeping late can result in difficult birth
- Believe childbirth causes a sudden loss of "yang forces," resulting in an imbalance in the body
- Believe hot foods, hot water, and warm air restore the yang forces
- Are attended to during labor by other women (usually patient's mother) — not the father of the baby
- Have stoic response to labor pain
- May prefer herbal medicine
- Restrict activity for 40 to 60 days postpartum
- Believe that colostrum is harmful (old, stale, dirty, poisonous, or contaminated) to baby so may delay breast-feeding until milk comes in

HISPANIC-AMERICANS

- View pregnancy as normal, healthy state
- May delay prenatal care
- Prefer a *patera* (midwife)
- Bring together mother's legs after childbirth to prevent air from entering uterus
- Are strongly influenced by the mother-in-law and mother during labor and birth and may listen to them rather than the husband
- View crying or shouting out during labor as acceptable
- May wear a religious necklace that's placed around the neonate's neck after birth
- Believe in hot and cold theory of disease and health
- Restricted to boiled milk and toasted tortillas for first 2 days after birth
- Must remain on bed rest for 3 days after birth
- Delay bathing for 14 days after childbirth
- Delay breast-feeding because colostrum is considered dirty and spoiled
- Don't circumcise male infants
- May place a bellyband on the neonate to prevent umbilical hernia

NATIVE AMERICANS

- View pregnancy as a normal, natural process
- May start prenatal care late
- Prefer a female birth attendant or a midwife
- May be assisted in birth by mother, father, or husband
- View birth as a family affair and may want entire family present
- May use herbs to promote uterine contractions, stop bleeding, or increase flow of breast milk
- Use cradle boards to carry baby and don't handle baby much
- May delay breast-feeding because colostrum is considered harmful and dirty
- May plan on taking the placenta home for burial

Cultural pain facts

Cultural and familial influences play a role in how a woman expresses or represses pain. These influences also determine whether she uses pharmacologic methods of pain relief. If her family views childbirth as a natural process or function for the female in the family unit, the woman is less likely to outwardly react to labor pains or require pharmacologic methods of pain relief.

Culture	Actions during pain
Filipino	■ Lie quietly during labor
Guatemalan	■ Express pain verbally
Hispanic	■ Are taught by their *pateras* (midwives) to endure pain and to keep their mouths closed during labor ■ Believe that to cry out would cause the uterus to rise and retard labor
Middle Eastern	■ Verbally expressive during labor ■ Often cry out and scream loudly ■ May refuse pain medication
Samoan	■ Believe they shouldn't express any pain verbally ■ Believe the pain must simply be endured ■ May refuse pain medication
Vietnamese, Laotian, and other Southeast Asian	■ Believe that crying out during labor is shameful ■ Believe that pain during labor must be endured

Fetal developmental milestones

The fetus typically achieves specific developmental milestones by the end of certain gestational weeks. By the end of the 4th week of gestation, for example, the fetus begins to show noticeable signs of growth in all areas assessed.

BY 4 WEEKS

- Head becomes prominent, accounting for about one-third of the entire embryo.
- Head is bent to such a degree that it appears as if it's touching the tail; embryo appears in a C shape.
- Heart appears in a rudimentary form as a bulge on the anterior surface.
- Eyes, ears, and nose appear in a rudimentary form.
- Nervous system begins to form.
- Extremities appear as buds.

BY 8 WEEKS

- Organ formation is complete.
- Head accounts for about one-half of the total mass.
- Heart is beating and has a septum and valves.
- Arms and legs are developed.
- Abdomen is large, with evidence of fetal intestines.
- Facial features are readily visible; eye folds are developed.
- Gestational sac is visible on ultrasound.

BY 12 WEEKS

- Nail beds are beginning to form on extremities; arms appear in normal proportions.
- Heartbeat can be heard using a Doppler ultrasound stethoscope.
- Kidney function is beginning; fetal urine may be present in amniotic fluid.
- Tooth buds are present.
- Placenta formation is complete with presence of fetal circulation.
- Gender is distinguishable with the visibility of external genitalia.

BY 16 WEEKS

- Fetal heart sounds are audible with stethoscope.
- Lanugo is present and well formed.
- Fetus demonstrates active swallowing of amniotic fluid.
- Fetal urine is present in amniotic fluid.
- The skeleton begins ossification.
- Intestines assume normal position in the abdomen.

BY 20 WEEKS

- Mother is able to feel spontaneous movements by the fetus.
- Hair begins to form, including eyebrows and scalp hair.
- Fetus demonstrates definite sleep and wake patterns.
- Brown fat begins to form.
- Sebum is produced by the sebaceous glands.
- Meconium is evident in the upper portion of the intestines.
- Lower extremities are fully formed.
- Vernix caseosa covers the skin.

BY 24 WEEKS

- Well-defined eyelashes and eyebrows are visible.
- Eyelids are open and pupils can react to light.
- Meconium may be present down to the rectum.
- Hearing is developing; the fetus begins to respond to sudden sounds.
- Lungs are producing surfactant.
- Passive antibody transfer from the mother begins (possibly as early as 20 weeks' gestation).

BY 28 WEEKS

- Surfactant appears in amniotic fluid.
- Alveoli in the lungs begin to mature.
- In the male, the testes start to move from the lower abdomen into the scrotal sac.
- Eyelids can open and close.
- Skin appears red.

BY 32 WEEKS

- Fetus begins to appear more rounded as more subcutaneous fat is deposited.
- Moro reflex is active.
- Fetus may assume a vertex or breech position in preparation for birth.
- Iron stores are beginning to develop.
- Fingernails increase in length, reaching the tips of the fingers.
- Vernix caseosa thickens.

BY 36 WEEKS

- Subcutaneous fat continues to be deposited.
- Soles of feet have one or two creases.
- Lanugo begins to decrease in amount.
- Fetus is storing additional glycogen, iron, carbohydrate, and calcium.
- Skin on the face and body begins to smooth.

BY 40 WEEKS

- Fetus begins to kick actively and forcefully, causing maternal discomfort.
- Vernix caseosa is fully formed.
- Soles of the feet demonstrate creases covering at least two-thirds of the surface.
- Conversion of fetal hemoglobin to adult hemoglobin begins.
- In the male, testes descend fully into the scrotal sac.

Fetal head diameters at term

The illustration below depicts three commonly used measurements of fetal head diameters. The measurements are averages for term neonates. Individual measurements vary with fetal size, attitude, and presentation.

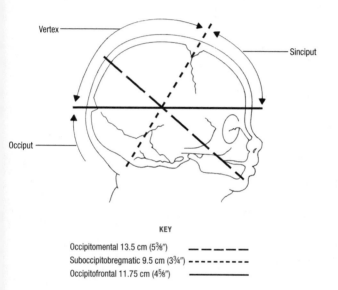

KEY

Occipitomental 13.5 cm (5⅜″) — — — — —
Suboccipitobregmatic 9.5 cm (3¾″) - - - - - - - -
Occipitofrontal 11.75 cm (4⅝″) —————

Fetal position abbreviations

The following abbreviations, organized according to variations in presentation, are used when documenting fetal position.

VERTEX PRESENTATION (OCCIPUT)

LOA, left occipitoanterior
LOP, left occipitoposterior
LOT, left occipitotransverse
ROA, right occipitoanterior
ROP, right occipitoposterior
ROT, right occipitotransverse

BREECH PRESENTATION (SACRUM)

LSaA, left sacroanterior
LSaP, left sacroposterior
LSaT, left sacrotransverse
RSaA, right sacroanterior
RSaP, right sacroposterior
RSaT, right sacrotransverse

FACE PRESENTATION (MENTUM)

LMA, left mentoanterior
LMP, left mentoposterior
LMT, left mentotransverse
RMA, right mentoanterior
RMP, right mentoposterior
RMT, right mentotransverse

SHOULDER PRESENTATION (ACROMION PROCESS)

LAA, left scapuloanterior
LAP, left scapuloposterior
RAA, right scapuloanterior
RAP, right scapuloposterior

Fetal presentation

Fetal presentation may be broadly classified as cephalic, breech, shoulder, or compound. Cephalic presentations occur in almost all deliveries. Of the remaining three, breech deliveries are most common.

CEPHALIC

In the cephalic, or head-down, presentation, the fetus's position may be classified by the presenting skull landmark: vertex, brow, sinciput, or mentum (chin).

VERTEX	BROW	SINCIPUT	MENTUM
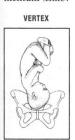	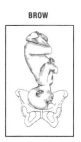	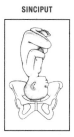	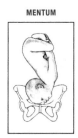

BREECH

In the breech, or head-up, presentation, the fetus's position may be classified as *complete*, where the knees and hips are flexed; *frank*, where the hips are flexed and knees remain straight; *footling*, where neither the thighs nor lower legs are flexed; and *incomplete*, where one or both hips remain extended and one or both feet or knees lie below the breech.

COMPLETE	FRANK	FOOTLING	INCOMPLETE
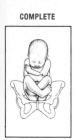	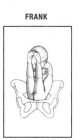	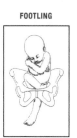	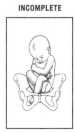

SHOULDER

Although a fetus may adopt one of several shoulder presentations, examination can't differentiate among them; thus, all transverse lies are considered shoulder presentations.

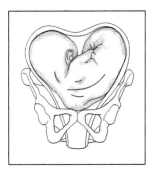

COMPOUND

In compound presentation, an extremity prolapses alongside the major presenting part so that two presenting parts appear in the pelvis at the same time.

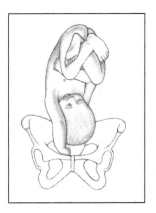

Health history and assessment findings

When performing the health history and assessment, look for the following findings to determine if a pregnant patient is at risk for complications.

DEMOGRAPHIC FACTORS

- Maternal age younger than 16 or older than 35
- Less than 11 years' education

LIFESTYLE

- Smoking (more than 10 cigarettes/day)
- Substance abuse
- Long commute to work
- Refusal to use seatbelts
- Alcohol consumption
- Heavy lifting or long periods of standing
- Lack of smoke detectors in home
- Unusual stress

OBSTETRIC HISTORY

- Infertility
- Grand multiparity
- Incompetent cervix
- Uterine or cervical anomaly
- Previous preterm labor or birth
- Previous cesarean birth
- Previous infant with macrosomia
- Two or more spontaneous or elective abortions
- Previous hydatidiform mole or choriocarcinoma
- Previous ectopic pregnancy
- Previous stillborn neonate or neonatal death
- Previous multiple gestation
- Previous prolonged labor
- Previous low-birth-weight infant
- Previous midforceps delivery
- Diethylstilbestrol exposure in utero

- Previous infant with neurologic deficit, birth injury, or congenital anomaly
- Less than 1 year since last pregnancy

MEDICAL HISTORY

- Cardiac disease
- Metabolic disease
- Renal disease
- Recent urinary tract infection or bacteriuria
- GI disorders
- Seizure disorders
- Family history of severe inherited disorders
- Surgery during pregnancy
- Emotional disorders or mental retardation
- Previous surgeries, particularly involving reproductive organs
- Pulmonary disease
- Endocrine disorders
- Hemoglobinopathies
- Sexually transmitted disease
- Chronic hypertension
- History of abnormal Papanicolaou smear
- Malignancy
- Reproductive tract anomalies

CURRENT OBSTETRIC STATUS

- Inadequate prenatal care
- Intrauterine growth–restricted fetus
- Large-for-gestational-age fetus
- Gestational hypertension
- Abnormal fetal surveillance tests
- Polyhydramnios
- Placenta previa
- Abnormal presentation
- Maternal anemia
- Weight gain of less than 10 lb (4.5 kg)
- Weight loss of more than 5 lb (2.3 kg)
- Overweight or underweight status
- Fetal or placental malformation

- Rh sensitization
- Preterm labor
- Multiple gestation
- Premature rupture of membranes
- Abruptio placentae
- Postdate pregnancy
- Fibroid tumors
- Fetal manipulation
- Cervical cerclage
- Maternal infection
- Poor immunization status
- Sexually transmitted infection

PSYCHOSOCIAL FACTORS

- Inadequate finances
- Social problems
- Adolescent
- Poor nutrition, poor housing
- More than two children at home with no additional support
- Lack of acceptance of pregnancy
- Attempt at or ideation of suicide
- No involvement of father of baby
- Minority status
- Parental occupation
- Inadequate support systems
- Dysfunctional grieving
- Psychiatric history

Neonatal laboratory values

This chart shows laboratory tests that may be ordered for neonates, including the normal ranges for full-term neonates. Note that ranges may vary among institutions. Because test results for preterm neonates usually reflect weight and gestational age, ranges for preterm neonates vary.

Test	Normal range
Blood	
Acid phosphatase	7.4 to 19.4 units/L
Albumin	3.6 to 5.4 g/dl
Alkaline phosphatase	40 to 300 units/L (1 week)
Alpha-fetoprotein	Up to 10 mg/L, with none detected after 21 days
Ammonia	90 to 150 mcg/dl
Amylase	0 to 1,000 IU/hour
Bicarbonate	20 to 26 mmol/L
Bilirubin, direct	< 0.5 mg/dl
Bilirubin, total	< 2.8 mg/dl (cord blood)
0 to 1 day	2.6 mg/dl (peripheral blood)
1 to 2 days	6 to 7 mg/dl (peripheral blood)
3 to 5 days	4 to 6 mg/dl (peripheral blood)
Bleeding time	2 minutes
Arterial blood gases	
pH	7.35 to 7.45
Partial pressure of arterial carbon dioxide (Paco$_2$)	35 to 45 mm Hg
Partial pressure of arterial oxygen (Pao$_2$)	50 to 90 mm Hg
Venous blood gases	
pH	7.35 to 7.45
Partial pressure of carbon dioxide (Pco$_2$)	41 to 51 mm Hg
Partial pressure of oxygen (Po$_2$)	20 to 49 mm Hg
Calcium, ionized	2.5 to 5 mg/dl
Calcium, total	7 to 12 mg/dl
Chloride	95 to 110 mEq/L
Clotting time (2 tube)	5 to 8 minutes
Creatine kinase	10 to 300 IU/L
Creatinine	0.3 to 1 mg/dl
Digoxin level	> 2 ng/ml possible; > 30 ng/ml probable
Fibrinogen	0.18 to 0.38 g/dl
Glucose	30 to 125 mg/dl
Glutamyltransferase	14 to 331 units/L
Hematocrit	52% to 58%
	53% (cord blood)
Hemoglobin	17 to 18.4 g/dl
	16.8 g/dl (cord blood)
Immunoglobulins, total	660 to 1,439 mg/dl
IgG	398 to 1,244 mg/dl
IgM	5 to 30 mg/dl
IgA	0 to 2.2 mg/dl
Iron	100 to 250 mcg/dl

Test	Normal range

Blood (continued)

Test	Normal range
Iron-binding capacity	100 to 400 mcg/dl
Lactate dehydrogenase	357 to 953 IU/L
Magnesium	1.5 to 2.5 mEq/L
Osmolality	270 to 294 mOsm/kg H_2O
Phenobarbital level	15 to 40 mcg/dl
Phosphorus	5 to 7.8 mg/dl (birth)
	4.9 to 8.9 mg/dl (7 days)
Platelets	100,000 to 300,000/µl
Potassium	4.5 to 6.8 mEq/L
Protein, total	4.6 to 7.4 g/dl
Prothrombin time	12 to 21 seconds
Partial thromboplastin time	40 to 80 seconds
Red blood cell (RBC) count	5.1 to 5.8 (1,000,000/µl)
Reticulocytes	3% to 7% (cord blood)
Sodium	136 to 143 mEq/L
Theophylline level	5 to 10 mcg/ml
Thyroid-stimulating hormone	< 7 microunits/ml
Thyroxine (T_4)	10.2 to 19 mcg/dl
Transaminase	
Glutamic-oxaloacetic (aspartate)	24 to 81 units/L
Glutamic-pyruvic (alanine)	10 to 33 units/L
Triglycerides	36 to 233 mg/dl
Urea nitrogen	5 to 25 mg/dl
White blood cell (WBC) count	18,000/µl
Eosinophils–basophils	3%
Immature WBCs	10%
Lymphocytes	30%
Monocytes	5%
Neutrophils	45%

Urine

Test	Normal range
Casts, WBCs	Present first 2 to 4 days
Osmolality	50 to 600 mOsm/kg
pH	5 to 7
Phenylketonuria	No color change
Protein	Present first 2 to 4 days
Specific gravity	1.006 to 1.008

Cerebrospinal fluid

Test	Normal range
Calcium	4.2 to 5.4 mg/dl
Cell count	0 to 15 WBCs/µl
	0 to 500 RBCs/µl*
Chloride	110 to 120 mg/L
Glucose	32 to 62 mg/dl
pH	7.33 to 7.42
Pressure	50 to 80 mm Hg
Protein	32 to 148 mg/dl
Sodium	130 to 165 mg/L
Specific gravity	1.007 to 1.009

* RBCs, red blood cells

Neonatal sutures and fontanels

NEONATAL SKULL SUPERIOR VIEW

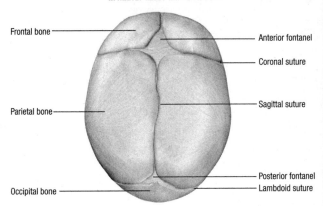

Frontal bone

Anterior fontanel

Coronal suture

Sagittal suture

Parietal bone

Posterior fontanel

Occipital bone

Lambdoid suture

Pregnancy abbreviation systems

Typically, an abbreviation system is used to summarize a woman's pregnancy information. Although many variations exist, a common abbreviation system consists of five letters — GTPAL.

Gravida = the number of pregnancies, including the present one.
Term = the total number of infants born at term or 37 or more weeks.
Preterm = the total number of infants born before 37 weeks.
Abortions = the total number of spontaneous or induced abortions.
Living = the total number of children currently living.

For example, if a woman pregnant once with twins delivers at 35 weeks' gestation and the neonates survive, the abbreviation that represents this information is "10202." During her next pregnancy, the abbreviation would be "20202."

An abbreviated but less informative version reflects only the *Gravida* and *Para* (the number of pregnancies that reached the age of viability — generally accepted to be 24 weeks, regardless of whether the babies were born alive or not).

In some cases, the number of abortions also may be included. For example, "G3, P2, Ab1" represents a woman who has been pregnant three times, who has had two deliveries after 24 weeks' gestation, and who has had one abortion. "G2, P1" represents a woman who has been pregnant two times and has delivered once after 24 weeks' gestation.

Pregnancy and nonpregnancy laboratory values

Test	Pregnant	Nonpregnant
Hemoglobin	11.5 to 14 g/dl	12 to 16 g/dl
Hematocrit	32% to 42%	36% to 48%
White blood cells	5,000 to 15,000/µl	4,500 to 10,000/µl
Neutrophils	60% ± 10%	60%
Lymphocytes	34% ± 10%	30%
Platelets	150,000 to 350,000/µl	150,000 to 350,000/µl
Serum calcium	7.8 to 9.3 mg/dl	8.4 to 10.2 mg/dl
Serum sodium	Increased retention	136 to 146 mmol/L
Serum chloride	Slight elevation	98 to 106 mmol/L
Serum iron	65 to 120 mcg/dl	75 to 150 mcg/dl
Fibrinogen	450 mg/dl	200 to 400 mg/dl
Red blood cells	1,500 to 1,900/mm^3	1,600/mm^3
Fasting blood glucose	Decreased	70 to 105 mg/dl
2-hour postprandial blood glucose	< 140 mg/dl (after a 100-g carbohydrate meal)	< 140 mg/dl
Blood urea nitrogen	Decreased	10 to 20 mg/dl
Serum creatinine	Decreased	0.5 to 1.1 mg/dl
Renal plasma flow	Increased by 25%	490 to 700 ml/minute
Glomerular filtration rate	Increased by 50%	88 to 128 ml/minute
Serum uric acid	Decreased	2 to 6.6 mg/dl
Erythrocyte sedimentation rate	Elevated during second and third trimesters	20 mm/hour
Prothrombin time	Decreased slightly	11 to 12.5 seconds
Partial thromboplastin time	Decreased slightly during pregnancy and again during second and third stages of labor (indicating clotting at placental site)	60 to 70 seconds

Pregnancy discomforts

This table lists common discomforts associated with pregnancy and suggestions for the patient on how to prevent and manage them.

Discomfort	Patient teaching
Urinary frequency	■ Void as necessary. ■ Avoid caffeine. ■ Perform Kegel exercises.
Fatigue	■ Try to get a full night's sleep. ■ Schedule a daily rest time. ■ Maintain good nutrition.
Breast tenderness	■ Wear a supportive bra.
Vaginal discharge	■ Wear cotton underwear. ■ Avoid tight-fitting pantyhose. ■ Bathe daily.
Backache	■ Avoid standing for long periods. ■ Apply local heat, such as a heating pad (set on low) or a hot water bottle. Make sure to place a towel between the heat source and the skin to prevent burning. ■ Stoop to lift objects — don't bend.
Round ligament pain	■ Slowly rise from a sitting position. ■ Bend forward to relieve pain. ■ Avoid twisting motions.
Constipation	■ Increase fiber intake in the diet. ■ Set a regular time for bowel movements. ■ Drink more fluids, including water and fruit juices (unless contraindicated). Avoid caffeinated drinks. ■ Rest on the left side with the hips and lower extremities elevated to provide better oxygenation to the placenta and fetus.
Hemorrhoids	■ Avoid constipation. ■ Apply witch hazel pads to the hemorrhoids. ■ Keep hemorrhoids reduced by using a well-lubricated gloved finger to push them gently inside the rectum; then tighten the rectal sphincter to support the hemorrhoids and contain them within the rectum. ■ Take sitz baths with warm water as often as needed to relieve discomfort.

(continued)

Discomfort	Patient teaching
Varicosities	■ Apply ice packs for reduction of swelling, if preferred over heat. ■ Walk regularly. ■ Rest with the feet elevated daily. ■ Avoid standing for long periods. ■ Avoid crossing the legs. ■ Avoid wearing constrictive knee-high stockings; wear support stockings instead.
Ankle edema	■ Avoid standing for long periods. ■ Rest with the feet elevated. ■ Avoid wearing garments that constrict the lower extremities.
Headache	■ Avoid eyestrain. ■ Rest with a cold cloth on the forehead.
Leg cramps	■ Straighten the leg and dorsiflex the ankle. ■ Avoid pointing the toes.

Pregnancy signs

This chart organizes signs of pregnancy into three categories: presumptive, probable, and positive.

Sign	Time from implantation (in weeks)	Other possible causes
Presumptive		
Breast changes (including feelings of tenderness, fullness, or tingling, and enlargement or darkening of areola)	2	■ Hyperprolactinemia induced by tranquilizers ■ Infection ■ Prolactin-secreting pituitary tumor ■ Pseudocyesis ■ Premenstrual syndrome
Nausea or vomiting upon arising	2	■ Gastric disorders ■ Infections ■ Psychological disorders, such as pseudocyesis and anorexia nervosa
Amenorrhea	2	■ Anovulation ■ Blocked endometrial cavity ■ Endocrine changes ■ Medications (phenothiazines) ■ Metabolic changes
Frequent urination	3	■ Emotional stress ■ Pelvic tumor ■ Renal disease ■ Urinary tract infection
Fatigue	12	■ Anemia ■ Chronic illness
Uterine enlargement (in which the uterus can be palpated over the symphysis pubis)	12	■ Ascites ■ Obesity ■ Uterine or pelvic tumor ■ Excessive flatus
Quickening (fetal movement felt by the woman)	18	■ Increased peristalsis ■ Cardiopulmonary disorders
Linea nigra (line of dark pigment on the abdomen)	24	■ Estrogen-progestin hormonal contraceptives ■ Obesity ■ Pelvic tumor
Melasma (dark pigment on the face)	24	■ Cardiopulmonary disorders ■ Estrogen-progestin hormonal contraceptives ■ Obesity ■ Pelvic tumor

(continued)

Sign	Time from implantation (in weeks)	Other possible causes
Presumptive (continued)		
Striae gravidarum (red streaks on the abdomen)	24	■ Cardiopulmonary disorders ■ Estrogen-progestin hormonal contraceptives ■ Obesity ■ Pelvic tumor
Probable		
Serum laboratory tests (revealing the presence of human chorionic gonadotropin [hCG] hormone)	1	■ Possible cross-reaction of luteinizing hormone (similar to hCG) in some pregnancy tests
Chadwick's sign (vagina changes color from pink to violet)	6	■ Hyperemia of cervix, vagina, or vulva
Goodell's sign (cervix softens)	6	■ Estrogen-progestin hormonal contraceptives
Hegar's sign (lower uterine segment softens)	6	■ Excessively soft uterine walls
Sonographic evidence of gestational sac (in which characteristic ring is evident)	6	■ None
Ballottement (fetus can be felt to rise against abdominal wall when lower uterine segment is tapped during bimanual examination)	16	■ Ascites ■ Uterine tumor or polyps
Braxton Hicks contractions (periodic uterine tightening)	20	■ Hematometra ■ Uterine tumor
Palpation of fetal outline (through abdomen)	20	■ Subserous uterine myoma
Positive		
Sonographic evidence of fetal outline	8	■ None
Fetal heart audible by Doppler ultrasound	10 to 12	■ None
Palpation of fetal movement (through abdomen)	20	■ None

RDAs for pregnant women

Energy and calorie requirements increase during pregnancy to create new tissue and to meet increased maternal metabolic needs. Nutrient requirements during pregnancy can be met by a diet that provides all of the essential nutrients, fiber, and energy in adequate amounts. The chart below gives recommended daily allowances (RDAs) for pregnant patients.

Calories	2,500 kcal
Protein	60 g
Fat-soluble vitamins	
Vitamin A	800 mcg
Vitamin D	10 mcg
Vitamin E	10 mcg
Water-soluble vitamins	
Ascorbic acid (vitamin C)	75 mg
Folic acid	400 mcg
Niacin	17 mg
Riboflavin	1.6 mg
Thiamine	1.5 mg
Vitamin B_6	2.2 mcg
Vitamin B_1	2.2 mcg
Minerals	
Calcium	1,200 mg
Phosphorus	1,200 mg
Iodine	175 mcg
Iron	30 mg
Zinc	15 mg

Weight conversion

Use this table to convert from pounds and ounces to grams when weighing neonates.

Ounces

Pounds	0	1	2	3	4	5	6
0	—	28	57	85	113	142	170
1	454	484	510	539	567	595	624
2	907	936	964	992	1021	1049	1077
3	1361	1389	1417	1446	1474	1503	1531
4	1814	1843	1871	1899	1928	1956	1984
5	2268	2296	2325	2353	2381	2410	2438
6	2722	2750	2778	2807	2835	2863	2892
7	3175	3203	3232	3260	3289	3317	3345
8	3629	3657	3685	3714	3742	3770	3799
9	4082	4111	4139	4167	4196	4224	4252
10	4536	4564	4593	4621	4649	4678	4706
11	4990	5018	5046	5075	5103	5131	5160
12	5443	5471	5500	5528	5557	5585	5613
13	5897	5925	5953	5982	6010	6038	6067
14	6350	6379	6407	6435	6464	6492	6520
15	6804	6832	6860	6889	6917	6945	6973

7	8	9	10	11	12	13	14	15
198	227	255	283	312	340	369	397	425
652	680	709	737	765	794	822	850	879
1106	1134	1162	1191	1219	1247	1276	1304	1332
1559	1588	1616	1644	1673	1701	1729	1758	1786
2013	2041	2070	2098	2126	2155	2183	2211	2240
2466	2495	2523	2551	2580	2608	2637	2665	2693
2920	2948	2977	3005	3033	3062	3090	3118	3147
3374	3402	3430	3459	3487	3515	3544	3572	3600
3827	3856	3884	3912	3941	3969	3997	4026	4054
4281	4309	4337	4366	4394	4423	4451	4479	4508
4734	4763	4791	4819	4848	4876	4904	4933	4961
5188	5216	5245	5273	5301	5330	5358	5386	5415
5642	5670	5698	5727	5755	5783	5812	5840	5868
6095	6123	6152	6180	6209	6237	6265	6294	6322
6549	6577	6605	6634	6662	6690	6719	6747	6776
7002	7030	7059	7087	7115	7144	7172	7201	7228

Selected references
Index

Selected references

Akert, J. "A New Generation of Contraceptives," *RN* 66(2):54-61, February 2003.

Association of Women's Health, Obstetric & Neonatal Nurses, *Women's Health Nursing—Towards Evidence Based Practice,* Philadelphia: W.B. Saunders Co., 2003.

Blackburn, S. *Maternal, Fetal and Neonatal Physiology,* 2nd ed.: *A Clinical Perspective.* Philadelphia: W.B. Saunders, Co., 2003.

Briggs, G.F., and Freeman, R.K. *Drugs in Pregnancy and Lactation: A Reference Guide to Fetal and Neonatal Risk,* 7th ed. Philadelphia: Lippincott Williams & Wilkins, 2005.

Buek, J.D., et al. "Successful External Cephalic Version after Amnioinfusion in a Patient with Preterm Premature Rupture of Membranes," *American Journal of Obstetrics and Gynecology* 192(6):2063-64, June 2005.

Callister, L.C., et al. "First-Time Mothers' Views of Breastfeeding Support from Nurses," *MCN, The American Journal of Maternal/Child Nursing* 28(1):10-15, January-February 2003.

Carr, D.B., et al. "A Sister's Risk: Family History as a Predictor of Preeclampsia," *American Journal of Obstetrics and Gynecology* 193(3 Pt 2):965-72, September 2005.

Fraser, W.D., et al. "Amnioinfusion for the Prevention of the Meconium Aspiration Syndrome," *New England Journal of Medicine* 353(9):909-17, September 2005.

Gomez, O., et al. "Uterine Artery Doppler at 11-14 Weeks of Gestation to Screen for Hypertensive Disorders and Associated Complications in an Unselected Population," *Ultrasound in Obstetrics & Gynecology* 26(5):490-94, October 2005.

Klossner, N.J., and Hatfield, N. *Introductory Maternity & Pediatric Nursing.* Philadelphia: Lippincott Williams & Wilkins, 2006.

Leifer, G. *Maternity Nursing: An Introductory Text*, 9th ed. Philadelphia: W.B. Saunders Co., 2005.

Morgan, G., and Hamilton, C. *Practice Guidelines for Obstetrics & Gynecology*, 2nd ed. Philadelphia: Lippincott Williams & Wilkins, 2003.

Murphy, P.A. "New Methods of Hormonal Contraception," *Nurse Practitioner* 28(2):11-21, February 2003.

Murray, S.S., and McKinney, E.S. *Foundations of Maternal-Newborn Nursing*, 4th ed. Philadelphia: W.B. Saunders Co., 2006.

Newman, M.G., et al. "Perinatal Outcomes in Preeclampsia that is Complicated by Massive Proteinuria," *American Journal of Obstetrics and Gynecology* 188(1):264-68, January 2003.

Pillitteri, A. *Maternal & Child Health Nursing*, 4th ed. Philadelphia: Lippincott Williams & Wilkins, 2003.

Scott, J.R., et al. *Danforth's Obstetrics and Gynecology*, 9th ed. Philadelphia: Lippincott Williams & Wilkins, 2003.

Speroff, L., and Darney, P. *A Clinical Guide for Contraception*, 4th ed. Philadelphia: Lippincott Williams & Wilkins, 2005.

Straight A's in Maternal-Neonatal Nursing. Philadelphia: Lippincott Williams & Wilkins, 2004.

Wong, D., et al. *Maternal Child Nursing Care*, 3rd ed. St. Louis: Mosby–Year Book, Inc., 2006.

Index

---

i refers to an illustration; t refers to a table.

i refers to an illustration; t refers to a table.

i refers to an illustration; t refers to a table.

i refers to an illustration; t refers to a table.

i refers to an illustration; t refers to a table.

i refers to an illustration; t refers to a table.

i refers to an illustration; t refers to a table.

---

i refers to an illustration; t refers to a table.

---

i refers to an illustration; t refers to a table.

---

i refers to an illustration; t refers to a table.

i refers to an illustration; t refers to a table.

---

i refers to an illustration; t refers to a table.

i refers to an illustration; t refers to a table.